Serena Lee Fazzolari is a food and lifestyle
blogger based in East London, UK. She founded
Vegans of LDN in 2014 as a resource to share
the best and most vegan-friendly places to
eat and drink around London, as well as other
ways to promote vegan living in the city. Her
blog and social media pages now serve London's
vegan community as a resource for where to
wine, dine and even go for a vegan-friendly
hair appointment — but the main focus will
always be Serena's first love: plant-based
food. *Vegan London* is her first book.

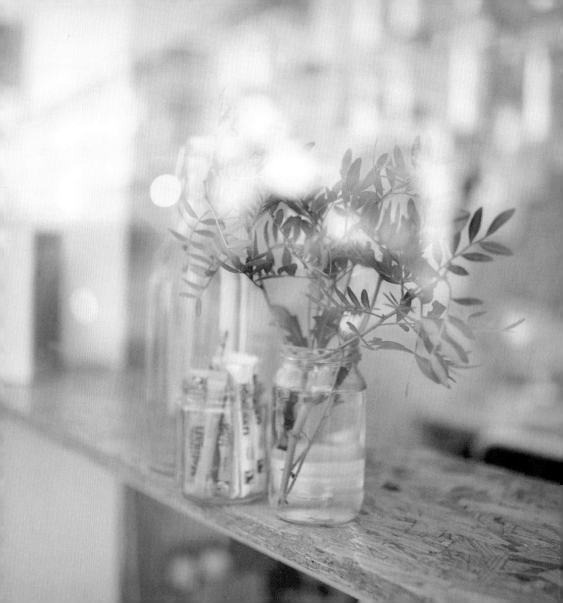

VEGAN LONDON

A GUIDE TO THE CAPITAL'S BEST CAFÉS, RESTAURANTS AND FOOD STORES

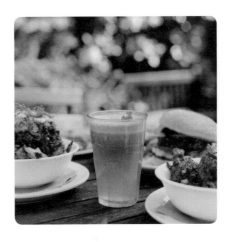

BY SERENA LEE

PHOTOGRAPHS BY JACK ORTON

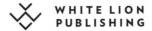

WHITE LION PUBLISHING

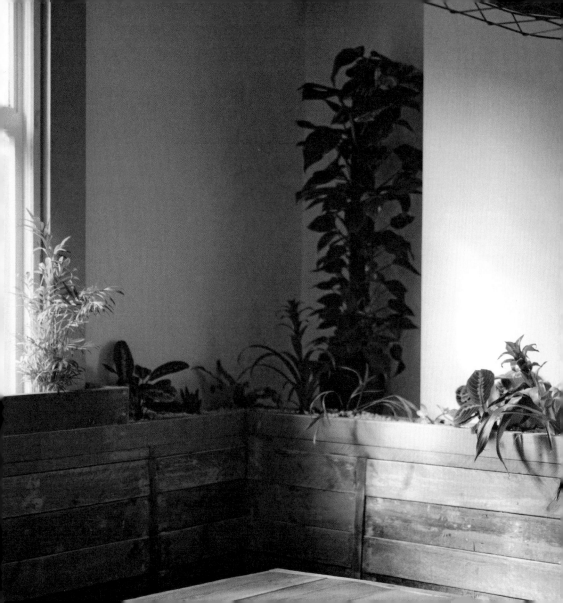

CONTENTS

INTRODUCTION

If you open a restaurant today without vegan options on the menu, you're missing a trick. Even some of the UK's most popular burger chains have U-turned in the last few years. One, for example, going from openly mocking vegans with adverts proclaiming that cows eat grass 'so you don't have to', to bringing out a vegan burger with a bean patty and jalapeño hummus. And it's no wonder - the number of vegans in the UK more than tripled between 2006 and 2016, with campaigns like 'Veganuary' helping thousands of people take the first steps towards an ethical vegan lifestyle. On top of this, plant-based diets are on the rise as the health-conscious strive to make plants the foundation of their meals, with more and more people also becoming conscious of how a plant-based diet can lower their carbon footprint.

As a result, the vegan scene in London is booming, with new fully vegan cafés, restaurants and pop-ups opening every month, and markets teeming with vegan street-food traders.

So whether you care about your health, the environment or animals (hopefully all three), use this book to navigate the city's plant-based scene, from its green juice to its deep-fried ice cream.

The restaurant world is ever-changing - recipes are adapted, restaurants move to different parts of town, street traders set up permanent locations. Check brand websites under each entry for current information so that you can enjoy the full *Vegan London* experience.

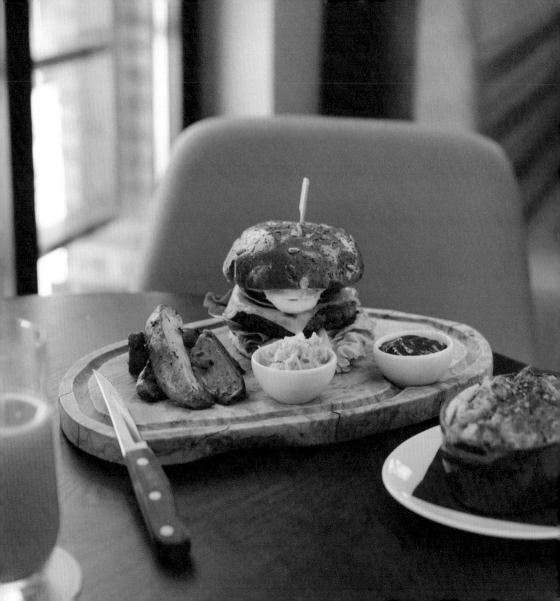

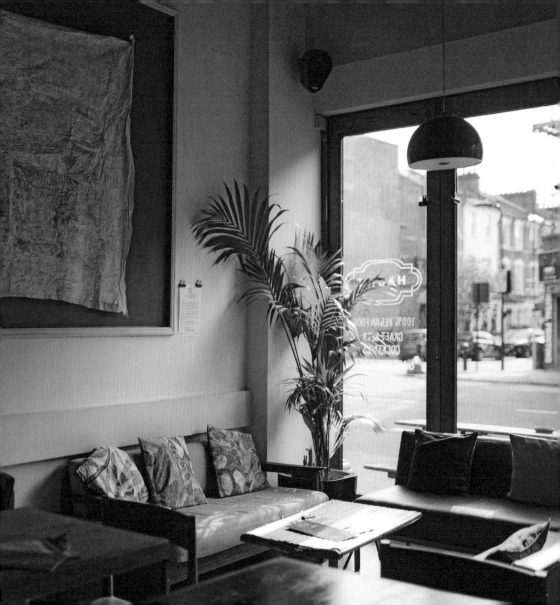

QUICK BITES

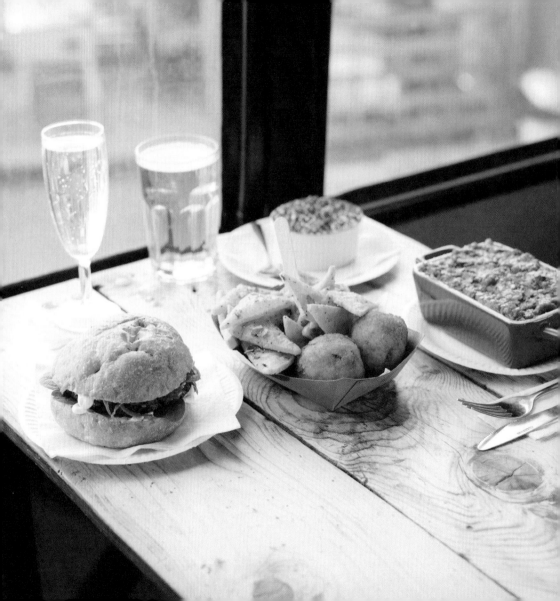

QUICK BITES

Vegan burgers, vegan pizzas and vegan fried chicken: long gone
are the days when a quick vegan meal meant a peanut-butter sandwich.
Market stalls are replacing their vegetarian options for more inclusive
vegan options, and pizzerias that don't yet offer vegan cheese will often
let you bring your own and put it in the oven for you. Fried food is at the
heart of grab-and-go culture, and the vegan world is no different –
you'll find breadcrumbed jackfruit as a substitute for pulled pork, moreish
arancini balls and mock kebab meat challenging the norms while saving
the animals. A lot of the food in this chapter you can eat with one hand,
so you can sign vegan petitions with the other. Or hold a coffee.
What you do with your free hand is up to you.

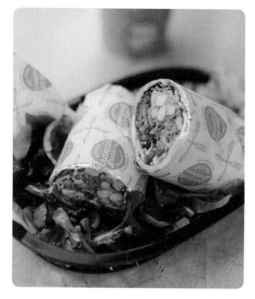
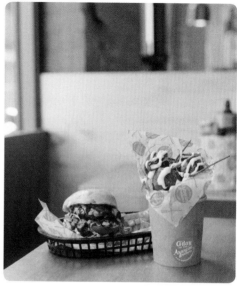

❖ ARANCINI BROTHERS 100% VEGAN

Crispy on the outside, chewy and gooey on the inside, Arancini Brothers base their food around one thing, and they do it to perfection. Rice grains are slow-cooked in herbs with garlic and onion, mixed with vegan cheese and then rolled by hand before being fried to a delicious golden hue. Big Dave and Little Dave started their arancini venture on Brick Lane, serving their food from a street-food stall, and eventually moved into a café in Kentish Town that soon became Arancini Brothers' first eatery. The two Daves learned the ways of arancini from Sicilian chefs while living and working in Australia and now they've transformed risotto balls into burger patties to combine the two popular foods into a superburger. Having gone fully vegan in 2018 across all three branches, the menu now extends to protein-packed stews as well as the old arancini favourites.

115A Kentish Town Road, NW1 8PB.
020 3583 2242
www.arancinibrothers.com
Camden Road Overground or Camden Town Tube.
Branches: Dalston E8 4AH, Old Street EC1V 9AE.

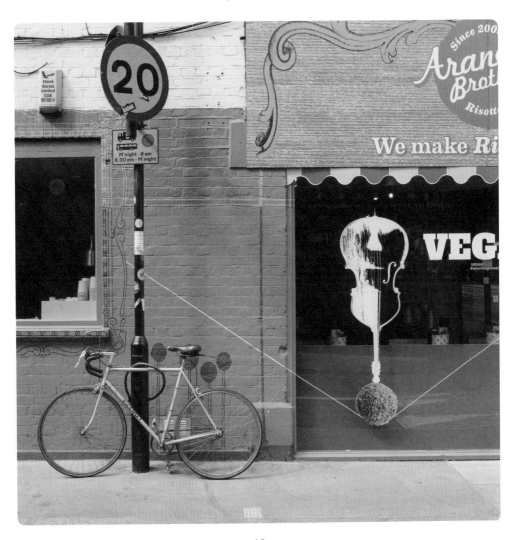

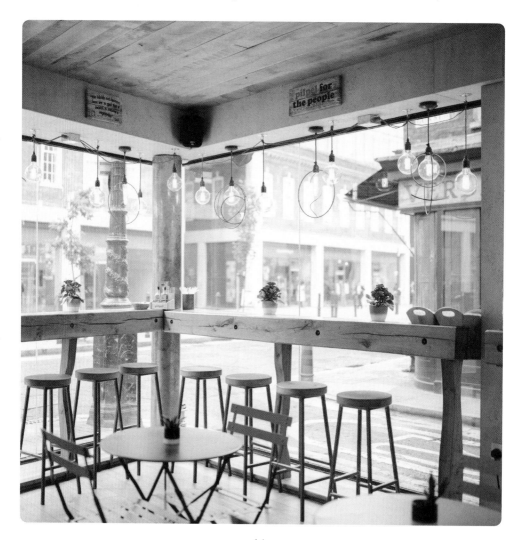

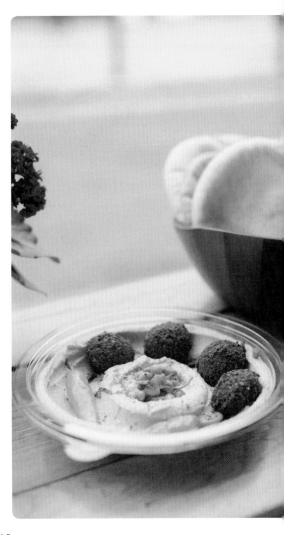

✦ PILPEL VEGAN-FRIENDLY

Pilpel first opened on Spitalfields' Brushfield Street
in 2009, inspired by Grandfather Zion's passion for
making flavoursome falafel with his secret recipe.
Founder Uri learned the ways of falafel while
working at his grandfather's stand in Israel
as a teenager, and decided to continue his legacy
by taking the recipe to London. Fast-forward a
decade and there are six sites across East and East-
Central London, each attracting queues of regulars
every day looking to get their fill of vegetarian
fast food. The falafel is what draws Londoners in,
with the perfect crispy balls offered in a pitta or
in a container, but the menu also includes hummus
bowls with salad and toppings. Load up with
aubergine, guacamole, sun-dried tomatoes and
pickled cucumbers. Uri's commitment to filling
falafel with only chickpeas, vegetables and spices
– with no added flour – makes Pilpel's the best
in town.

—

38 Brushfield Street, E1 6AT.
020 7952 5768
www.pilpel.co.uk
Liverpool Street Tube.
Branches: Aldgate E1 8PX, Fleet Street EC4M 3BY,
Lime Street EC3V 1PL, Spitalfields Market E1 6EW,
St Paul's EC4M 7DZ.

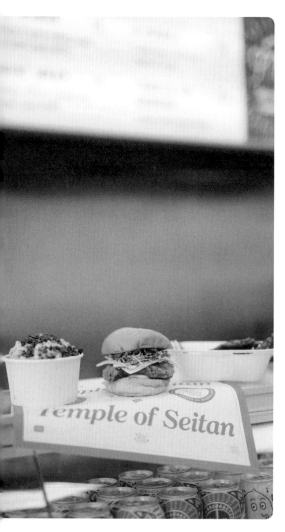

❧ TEMPLE OF SEITAN 100% VEGAN

At London's first vegan fried 'chicken' shop, queues can often reach around the corner – much to the frustration of Hackney Meat Centre just next door. Temple of Seitan began serving their wheat-based chicken alternative at markets, launching their first eatery in early 2017. In an area full of traditional fried chicken and fast-food takeaways, founding branch Temple of Hackney is a firm favourite among locals and meat-eaters alike and, while there's no seating inside, it doesn't really matter when vegan fried 'chicken' tastes this good. Take your pick between vegan chicken wings and popcorn chicken or keep it simple with chicken fillets and chips. Temple of Hackney (or their sister branch, Temple of Camden) should be high up on your list of places to take your non-vegan friends. Bet them that they'll be pleasantly surprised and enjoy the moreish crunch of real fast food.

—

10 Morning Lane, E9 6NA.
www.templeofseitan.co.uk
Hackney Central Overground.
Siblings: Temple of Camden N1C 4PF.

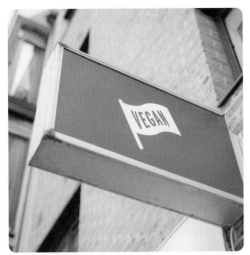

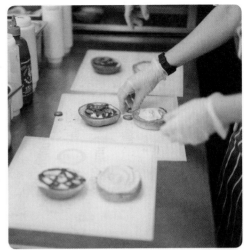

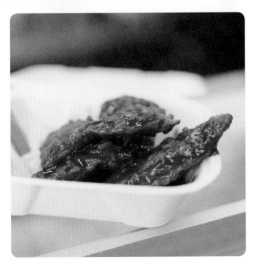

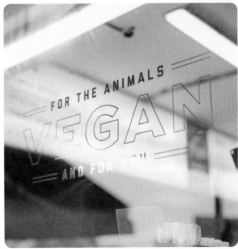

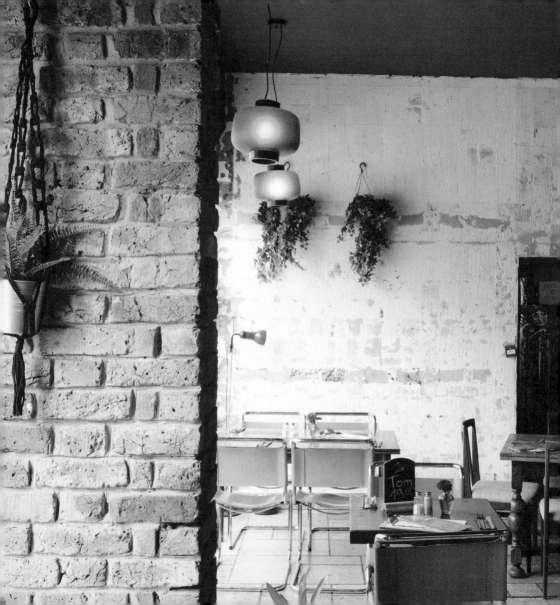

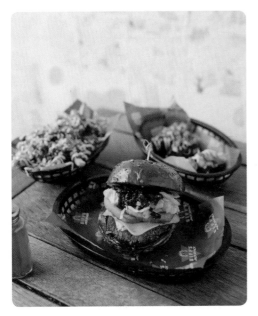

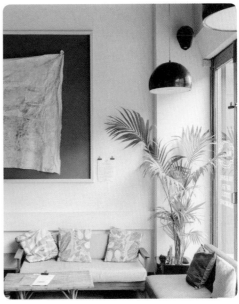

✧ BIFF'S JACK SHACK <u>100% VEGAN</u>

An ideal restaurant to take your non-vegan friends, Biff's Jack Shack serves some of the dirtiest vegan junk food in London. Situated within Boxpark in Shoreditch, Biff's whole menu is vegan. You'll be surprised at how indulgent jackfruit can be when crafted into burger patties through braising, a double-dip in panko crumb and a good old fry. Choose from burger options like The Father Jack with smoky 'bacun' jam, bourbon barbecue sauce, smoked vegan cheese, iceberg lettuce and onion rings, and the equally stacked Jacksu with katsu sauce, Japanese pickles, crisp lettuce and a tempura broccoli floret. If you have room for more, try the jackfruit 'wingz', complete with a sugar cane 'bone' for an ethical meat-like experience.

It's one of your five-a-day, but not as you know it.

—

49, Boxpark Shoreditch, 2-10 Bethnal Green Road, E1 6GY.
07717 174 971
www.biffsjackshack.com
Shoreditch High Street Overground.
Branches: Walthamstow, E17 9NJ.

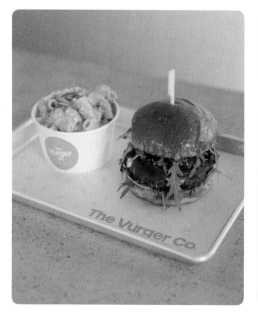

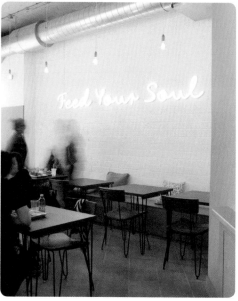

❖ THE VURGER CO. <u>100% VEGAN</u>

Having started out as a pop-up, The Vurger Co. launched a hugely successful crowdfunding campaign in 2017 that helped them open a site not far from Shoreditch High Street station, where they've become popular with locals as well as pulling in hoards of vegans from further afield. A company proud to be revolutionising fast food by taking vegetables, seeds, nuts, grains and legumes and forming them into some of the best burgers in East London, everything at The Vurger Co. is 100 percent vegan, from the patties to the mac 'n'

cheese to the housemade shakes (try the banana caramel for some sweet, guilt-free hydration). There are four burgers on the menu, including the MLT with borlotti beans, roasted mushrooms and a tomato and walnut pesto. Sink your teeth into these alongside a glass of vegan beer, cider or wine before heading out for the evening on Brick Lane.

——

Unit 9, Avant Garde Building, 6 Richmix Square, Cygnet Street, E1 6LD.

www.thevurgerco.com

Shoreditch High Street Overground.

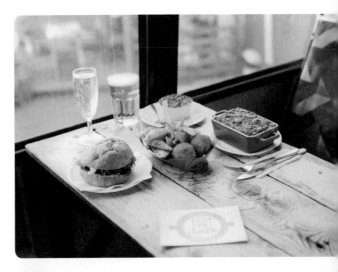

✤ JUSTFAB 100% VEGAN

Inspired by the Sicilian street-food scene, and with an urge to share with the world his own mamma's incredible vegan cooking, Fabio Pironti set up his own street-food bus in London, feeding crowds at festivals before settling in Hackney in 2015. Mamma Myra even moved from Sicily to perfect the menu, and the result is a true culinary gem. JustFaB is a vegan eatery with a difference – situated within a converted red, double-decker London bus with upstairs seating and home-cooked food, they serve vegan twists on classic Italian dishes, including lasagna, panelle, arancini filled with mushroom and made without dairy, and an amazing tiramisu. You can eat in, on top of the bus, or you can get it to take away (they also deliver locally). Whether you're vegan or just a lover of Italian food, you won't be disappointed with JustFaB's authentic 'veg-Italian' food.

----

455 Hackney Road, London E2 9DY.
07414 917 637
www.just-fab.org
Cambridge Heath Overground.

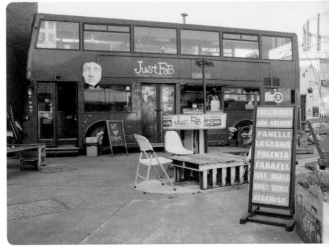

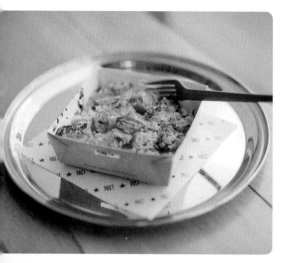

✤ VEGGIE PRET <u>VEGAN-FRIENDLY</u>

The people spoke, and internationally-renowned Pret a Manger listened – having morphed their Broadwick Street site into a vegetarian-only eatery in 2016 as a month-long pop-up, Veggie Pret was such a successful experiment that the chain turned one of their Shoreditch branches into a Veggie Pret too, and subsequently also opened up a new, veggie-since-inception store at Exmouth Market. There are plenty of treats on offer at Veggie Pret, with a refreshingly regular rotation of new foods making their way onto the shelves. Look out for new vegan menu items on Pret's social media – popular products have included Mac and Greens, the Dark chocolate and Almond-butter Cookie and their Mango Chia Pot. There's something for everyone at Veggie Pret – and their omnipresence across London means there's always an affordable vegan option nearby, with the familiarity and quality of the Pret a Manger brand.

---

35 Broadwick Street, W1F 0DH.

020 7932 5274

www.pret.co.uk/en-gb/veggie-pret

Oxford Circus or Piccadilly Circus Tube.

Branches: Great Eastern Street, EC2A 3QD,
Exmouth Market, EC1R 4QD.

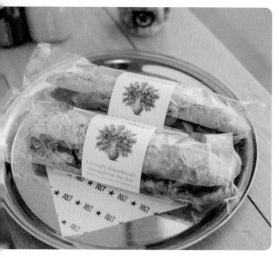

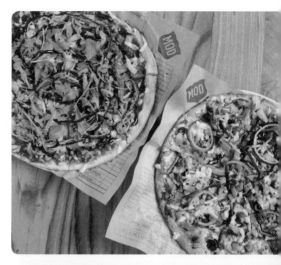

❖ MOD PIZZA VEGAN-FRIENDLY

Known for its build-your-own pizza concept,
MOD is a non-vegan pizza chain with its doors
wide open to vegan diners – a welcome notion
in Leicester Square where, at a lot of popular
restaurants, vegans remain an afterthought.
Reassuringly, MOD Pizza encourages vegans to let
the server know of dietary requirements so that
different gloves can be worn, and so that the pizza
can be prepared in a specific area to try and avoid
cross-contamination with other ingredients. The
pizza dough at MOD is free from animal products
naturally, and there's a wide range of veggie
toppings to choose from. Start with a red sauce or
barbecue sauce, and then add on everything from
roasted sweetcorn to black olives, pineapple and
chickpeas. On top of this, if you're laying off the
bread, you can load up a salad and drizzle it with
fig glaze or sriracha.

17–18 Irving Street, WC2H 7AT.
020 7839 2714
www.modpizza.co.uk
Leicester Square Tube.

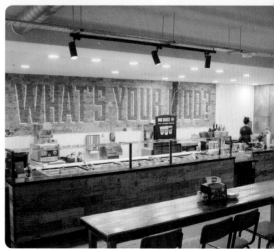

23

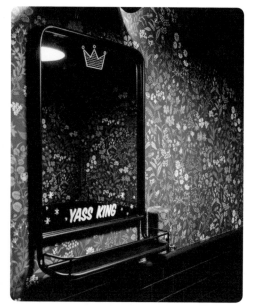

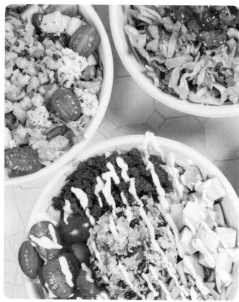

❖ BY CHLOE. 100% VEGAN

Fast-casual vegan restaurant by CHLOE. first opened in New York in 2015, and has since gained a huge following for its Instagrammable interior as well as its soul-satisfying plant-based food. Crossing the pond in early 2018 to open a restaurant in Covent Garden, you can delight in eating your smashed-avocado toast under neon lights proclaiming 'Guac save the Queen' before getting involved with a steaming peanut-butter hot cocoa. by CHLOE. also serve up crispy tofu fish 'n' chips, a pea 'n' ham soup and a shepherd's pie with ground seitan, mashed potato and beet ketchup. Food is ordered at the counter and served on trays, giving vegans everything they want from a fast-food experience, just without the meat. If you have non-vegan friends, convince them to come for the aesthetic and they'll be converted in no time.

Drury House, 34–43 Russell Street, WC2B 5HA.
www.eatbychloe.com
Covent Garden Tube.
Branches: Tower Bridge, SE1 2SD.

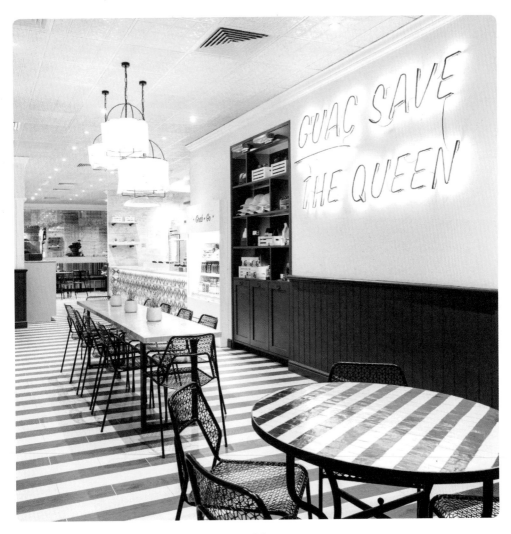

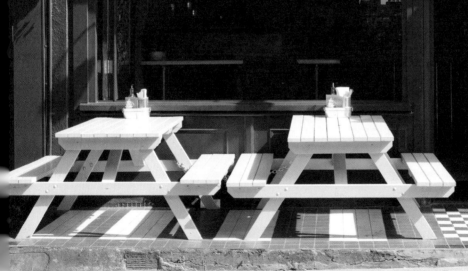

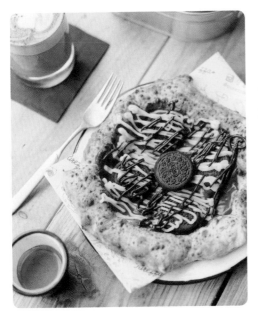

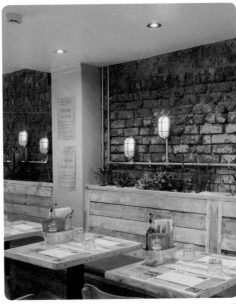

❖ PUREZZA 100% VEGAN

With ten drool-worthy sourdough pizzas on the menu, plus calzone, raw pizza and lasagna, you'll need to schedule in repeat visits to Purezza in order to get over any fear of missing out on their incredible Italian food. The pizzeria proved so popular in Brighton that Purezza opened a branch in Camden, also serving up smoothies, coffees, beer, wine and cocktails. Having spent two years perfecting their mozzarella recipe using brown rice – resulting in a cheese with half the calories and fat compared with traditional mozzarella – the team is dedicated to feeding Londoners nothing but the best, offering up pizzas like the Couch Potato (smoked mozzarella, aubergine, potatoes, basil and seitan) and the Cheesus made with four types of vegan cheese. Feast on these with a side of cheesy dough balls and finish with a creamy, hazelnutty Oreo pizza. Pure gluttony.

—

43 Parkway, NW1 7PN.
020 3884 0078
www.purezza.co.uk
Camden Town Tube.

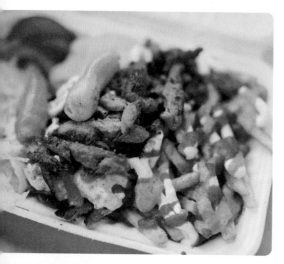

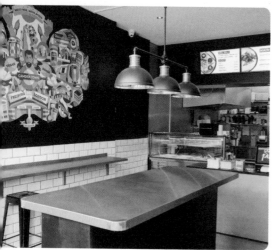

✤ WHAT THE PITTA 100% VEGAN

Offering a high-quality, plant-based alternative to one of the UK's junk food favourites – the humble döner kebab – What The Pitta serve up juicy wraps packed to the brim with non-GMO soya chunks, salad, vegan tzatziki, homemade hummus and even freshly made bread (also available as a couscous box). Attracting locals and tourists alike at their ever-busy Boxpark eatery in Shoreditch, What The Pitta also make vegan *lamacun* – Turkish pizza – topped with minced soya, onions, minced vegetables and herbs. Finish your hearty meal with a satisfyingly sweet vegan baklava, so sticky it's almost dripping. This is one of the top spots to take your non-vegan friends and challenge their perception of what it means to eat vegan – and they've now also opened branches in Boxpark Croydon and Camden, so if you're not in East London you can still eat your fill of vegan Turkish food.

—

Unit 52, Boxpark Shoreditch, 2–10 Bethnal Green Road, E1 6GY.
www.whatthepitta.com
Shoreditch High Street Overground or Liverpool Street Tube/rail.
Branches: Camden NW1 0AG, Croydon CR0 1LD.

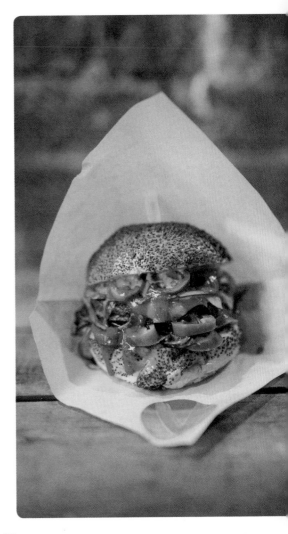

✛ BIG V <u>100% VEGAN</u>

Juicy patties, bacon, cheddar, smoked cheese, chipotle mayo, poppy-seed brioche buns – there's nothing Big V can't veganise, and convincingly too. Since setting up their original market stall at Borough Market, they've made a name for themselves as a mouth-watering, plant-based alternative to the junk food options spilling over at markets London-wide. Attracting hordes of hungry market-goers wherever they're cooking, these are classic burger flavours with a healthy spin, and you can even get a V Bowl with a patty, a dressed salad and hummus if you don't fancy a bun. Try the Holy Smoke with smoked cheese, smoky house barbecue sauce, maple 'facon' (vegan bacon), chipotle mayo and caramelised onions – or, for a taste of all the fillings, grab a Big V Facon Cheeseburger with burger sauce, tomato relish, pickles, red onion and vegan cheddar. Whatever you choose, you won't be left hungry.

Market trader (check website for current locations)
www.bigvlondon.co.uk

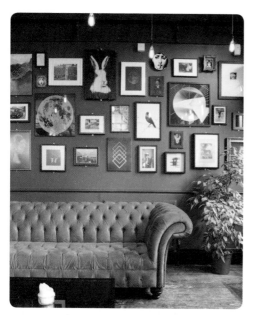
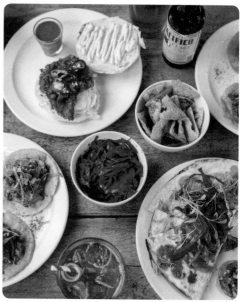

✤ CLUB MEXICANA <u>100% VEGAN</u>

This is street food how it's meant to be done: deep-fried, spicy and loaded. Club Mexicana serve Mexican-inspired dishes that are all vegan, with a side of disco vibes under neon lights. Start your meal with vegan cheese sticks, fried in breadcrumbs, they break into a gooey, stringy centre that will strip your veggie friend of their 'can't give up cheese' line when debating going fully vegan. Next up, try the Mexicana Hot Nachos or the Pulled Jackfruit Burrito with guacamole, pink pickled onion and salted chillies.

If it's your lucky day, there might even be deep-fried Mexican ice cream on the menu for dessert. A favourite at markets across London, keep up with current locations on their website – you'll find their tofish tacos all over town if you know where to look. They also have a long-term residency at The Spread Eagle vegan pub on Homerton High Street.

———

The Spread Eagle, 224 Homerton High Street, E9 6AS.
www.clubmexicana.com
Homerton Overground.

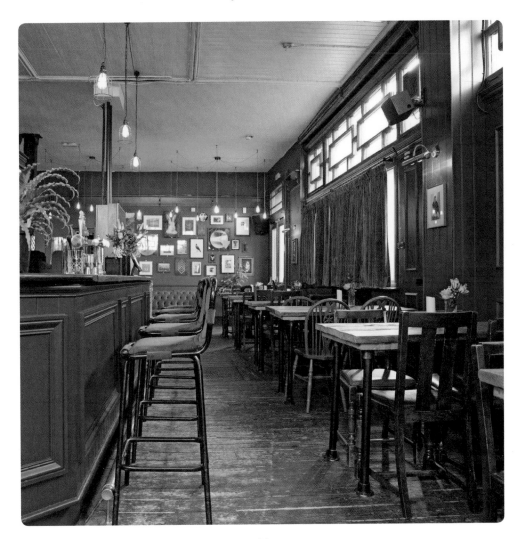

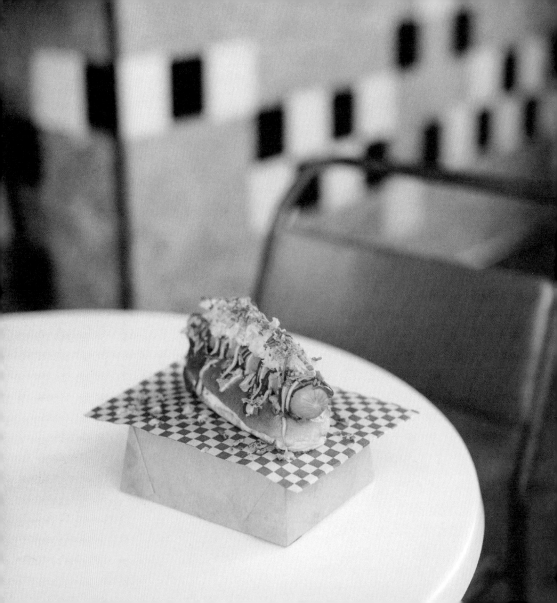

GOING GLOBAL

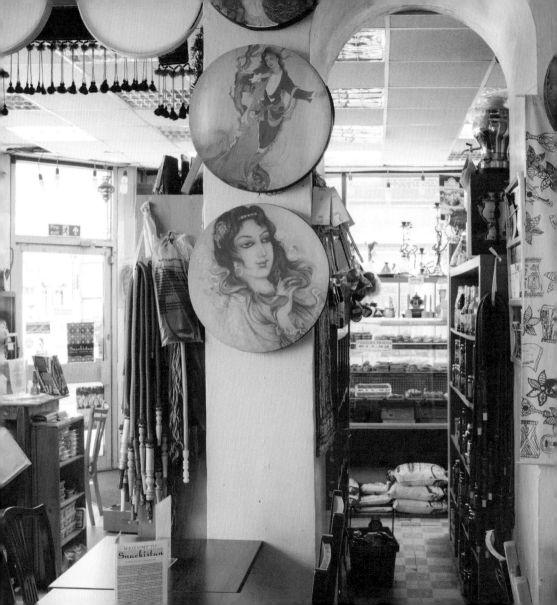

GOING GLOBAL

London is a tapestry rich in culture, with fascinating history and diversity – and all of this is reflected in its food. With plant foods traditionally being the staple of so many cuisines across the world, it's no surprise that the growing vegan movement has been met with an increase in global vegan dishes from both pre-existing restaurants and new independent vegan traders. London now has a melting pot of the original and the reinvented – pulses and grains at one restaurant, convincing vegan 'prawns' at another, and often both under one roof. From Ethiopian to Persian to Vietnamese, whatever your appetite calls for, you'll find it at a local vegan café, nestled in a broader restaurant menu or proudly presented at a vegan street-food stall at one of London's famous food markets.

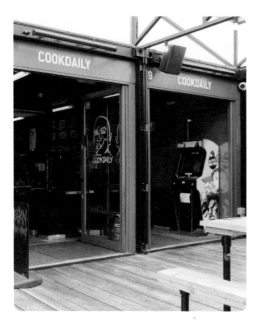

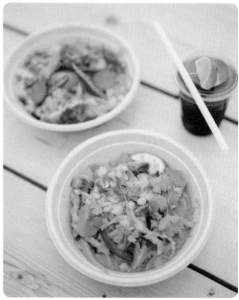

✤ COOKDAILY <u>100% VEGAN</u>

Smashing the stereotype that veganism is only for health bloggers and hippies, CookDaily draws in diverse crowds with its unapologetic approach to vegan food. Chef and founder King's mission in life is to make more people vegan and, since opening up his first CookDaily branch in 2015, he's served up plant-based bowls to thousands – even encouraging unsuspecting teens to try vegan food, drawn in by the frequent presence of their favourite celebrities at the restaurant. You'll have sixteen dishes to choose from, representing different cuisines from around the world with a heavy Southeast Asian influence, as King's heritage is from Laos. Favourites include the House Pad Thai with egg-style tofu, the Jerk and the High Grade, a sweet-and-sour smoky barbecue stir-fry with hemp-seed crumbles.

Arch 358 Westgate St, E8 3RN.
07498 563 168
www.cookdaily.co.uk
London Fields Overground.

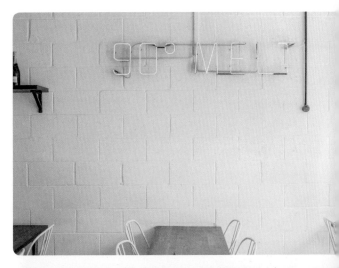

❖ 90 DEGREE MELT <u>VEGAN-FRIENDLY</u>

Comfort food is the name of the game at 90 Degree Melt. The East London American-style diner caters specifically towards a vegetarian market and has spent time honing their sustainable and responsibly sourced vegan menu. Known for their vegan cheese melted sandwiches, the restaurant is one of the best places in the area to get your weekly hit of rich, gooey, vegan cheese (there's also dairy on the menu, so order diligently). Combine the food with the modest dining area, friendly staff and an open kitchen in an unassuming part of Stepney, and 90 Degree Melt instantly becomes a classic local spot. The best time to visit 90 Degree Melt? Put it on your brunch list – they have solid options, from their vegan chilli to their tofu shakshuka served with guacamole. It's the perfect way to kick off the weekend.

—

235 Mile End Road, E1 4AA.
020 3754 5711
www.90degreemelt.co.uk
Stepney Green Tube.

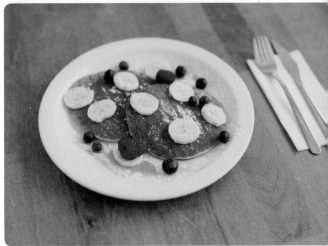

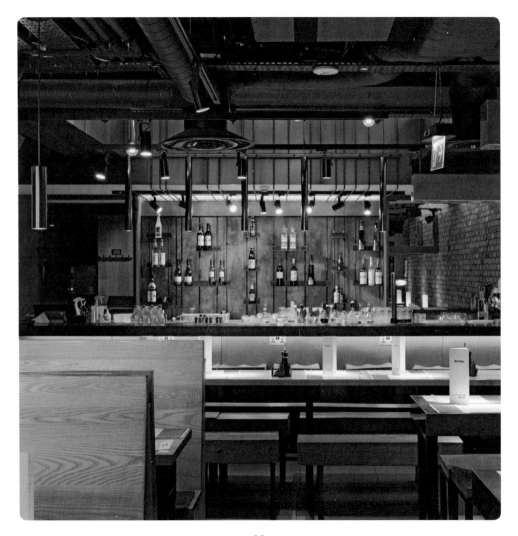

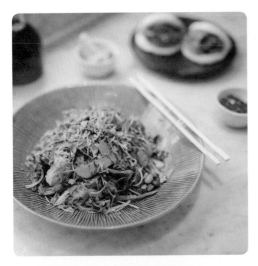

❖ WAGAMAMA VEGAN-FRIENDLY

A household name more present in London than any other city, you'll never be too far from great ramen with Wagamama. In line with its philosophy of kaizen, meaning 'good change' in Japanese, the restaurant chain brought out a separate vegan and vegetarian menu in 2017 – of the 29 dishes, around half are suitable for vegans, leaving plant-based diners spoilt for choice. Including listings of all the vegan-friendly drinks on offer, you can relax in the knowledge that even the Kansho lime and ginger pale ale is good to drink. Menu highlights include the ever-popular Yasai Gyoza and the Vegatsu – a seitan and panko breadcrumb re-imagination of Wagamama's classic katsu curry. For dessert, choose from refreshing sorbets of pink guava and passion fruit served with fresh mint. All dishes are freshly prepared and brought to the table as soon as they're ready for a laid-back dining experience.

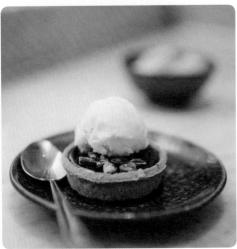

81 Dean Street, W1P 3HP.
020 3198 2984
www.wagamama.com
Tottenham Court Road Tube.
Branches: Camden NW1 7BW, London Bridge SE1 9BU, plus thirty other locations across London.

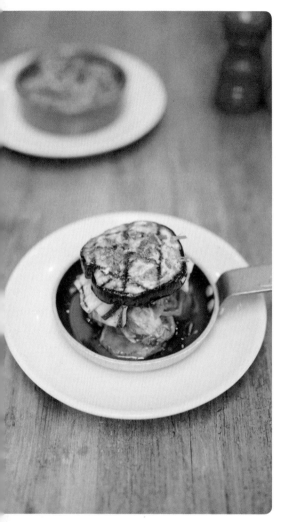

✤ THE REAL GREEK VEGAN-FRIENDLY

With ten locations across London including Soho, Spitalfields and both Westfield malls, The Real Greek is the capital's best option for vegan Grecian food. While the restaurant serves meat, there's a whole menu inspired by traditional vegan diets common in Greece, making use of fresh ingredients like vine leaves and lentils. Choose from an impressive thirty dishes, including vegan moussaka with a slow-cooked jackfruit mix, courgette, aubergine and cinnamon, and the Santorini Fava with yellow lentils, onion and fennel. The Bankside branch is perfect for a bite to eat after a visit to the Tate Modern, and there's Greek music performed every Friday and Saturday evening. If you'd prefer to enjoy your food outdoors, the Dulwich Village restaurant houses an outdoor space when the weather is agreeable – if not, it's also a treat to dine inside among the fresh, Santorini-inspired blue and white interior.

—

Units 1&2 Riverside House, 2A Southwark
Bridge Road, SE1 9HA.
020 7620 0162
www.therealgreek.com
Mansion House or London Bridge Tube.
Branches: Dulwich SE21 7AQ, Covent Garden
WC2E 9JE, plus seven more locations across London.

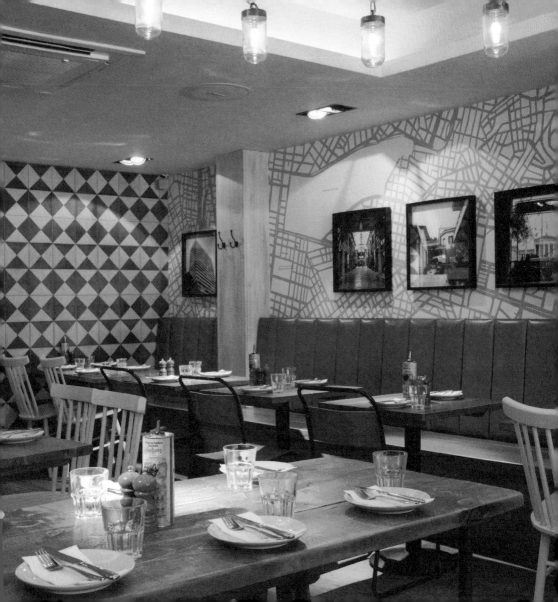

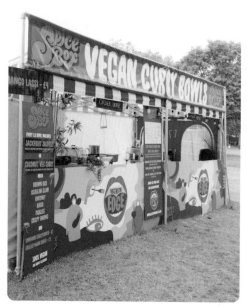

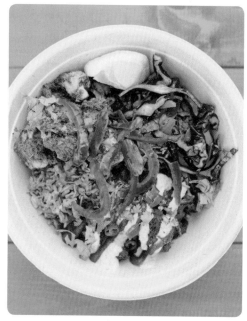

✤ SPICEBOX 100% VEGAN

SpiceBox was born from a love for Indian food in all its glory. London is full of great-quality Indian cuisine, but SpiceBox was the first market trader to offer grab-and-go, fully vegan Indian food that saves diners asking questions about ghee and paneer in vegetarian dishes. Starting out serving deliveries from founder Grace's home, SpiceBox soon grew to open a kiosk site at KERB Camden in October 2017, garnering heaps of press attention in the process – their tarka dhal was even awarded Best Dhal in the British Dhal Championships 2018. With dishes like the Cauli Tikka Masala in a creamy curry sauce and the Sweet Potato Salan on the menu, SpiceBox is a healthier alternative to a Friday night curry.

—

58 Hoe Street, Walthamstow E17 4PG.
0208 521 0906
www.eatspicebox.co.uk
Walthamstow Central Tube.

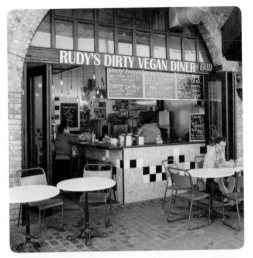

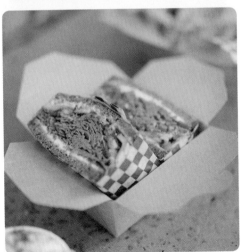

✛ RUDY'S DIRTY VEGAN DINER <u>100% VEGAN</u>

Now that Rudy's is in town, it feels as though Camden has been waiting for a dirty vegan diner for years. It's difficult to picture all-American comfort food without stacks of meat and cheese spilling from the sides, but Ruth (AKA Rudy) shatters misconceptions with diner dishes that taste just like the originals. Find the restaurant in the west of Camden Market, spicing up the Camden vegan food scene with loaded jalapeño nachos, the Dirty Burger and more. One of Rudy's most popular dishes is the reuben sandwich on rye bread, with vegan pastrami, onions, vegan cream cheese and sauerkraut — order with a side of Dirty Fries. Being ethical vegans, the Rudy's team strive to bring true comfort food to the masses, and bustling Camden is one of the best places to do it from. Bring your dog (Rudy's is pooch-friendly), your appetite and your highest expectations.

Unit 739, Camden Stables Market, NW1 8AH.
www.facebook.com/rudysDVD
Camden Town Tube.

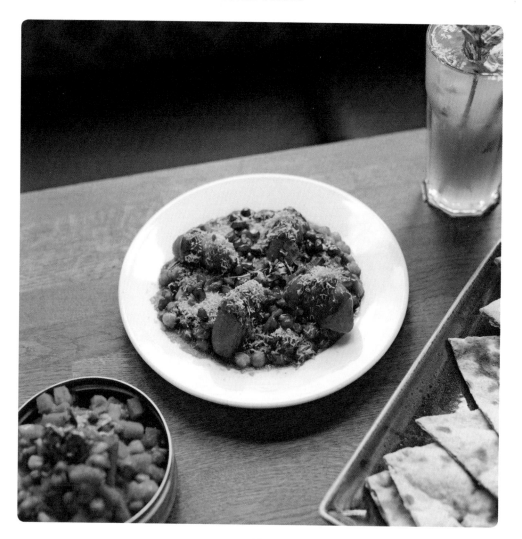

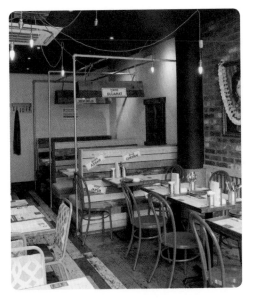

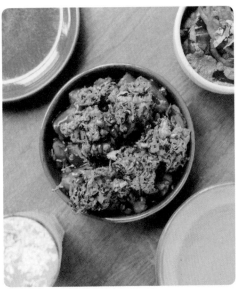

❖ CHAI NAASTO <u>VEGAN-FRIENDLY</u>

Chai Naasto have three restaurants across London, but the Harrow branch takes the crown when it comes to vegan options – the whole menu is vegetarian and you'll be spoilt for choice with plant-based food. With a unique and endearing back-story involving three brothers paying homage to their Nani's heritage and travels, you'll find Indian food with a twist at Chai Naasto, folding in flavours from India, Somalia, Saudi Arabia and the UK. On the Chaat Street section of the menu, you'll find roadside snacks like the Spicy Peanut and Potato Mash with pomegranate and green chutney, and the Pani Puri Shots – crisp wheat balls stuffed with spicy potato and a sweet-and-sour tamarind reduction. Or try the Chole and Kale Peshawari – chickpeas seasoned with chana masala and tossed in onion gravy. Nani's grandsons have done her proud.

---

242 Streatfield Road, HA3 9BX.
020 8204 4660
www.chai-naasto.co.uk
Queensbury Tube.
Branches: Beckenham BR3 3LD, Hammersmith W6 0NQ.

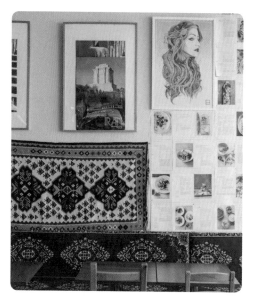
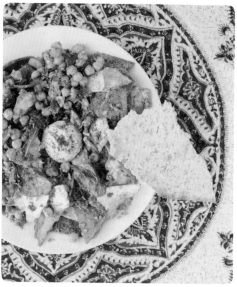

✿ PERSEPOLIS <u>VEGAN-FRIENDLY</u>

Snackistan at Persepolis Café offers a vegetarian menu with delicious vegan Persian options. After perusing the vegan-friendly pastry counter and the rest of the goods stocked in Persepolis's corner shop (within which the café is situated), enjoy a candlelit dinner, sharing dishes from their meze selection. Great things come from their modest kitchen, and you'll treasure Persepolis for its unforgettable people as well as its food – owner Sally is famous for her character as much as she is for her cookbooks. There's scrambled tofu with fried harissa plantain, okra and mushrooms and some of Peckham's most-loved hot drinks, including the saffron tea with *nabat* – 'posh crystallised ginger' – and the fragrant Persian tea with cardamom. The tasting/party menu is a must for first-timers – allowing you to spend less time pondering which intriguing dish to order and more time tucking into Persian delights.

—

28–30 Peckham High Street, SE15 5DT.
020 7639 8007
www.foratasteofpersia.co.uk
Peckham Rye Overground.

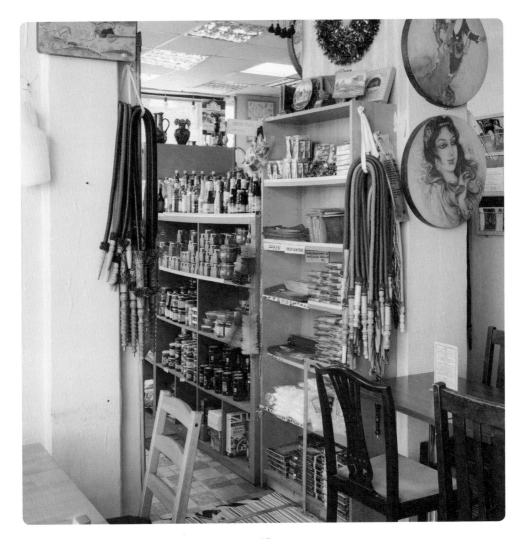

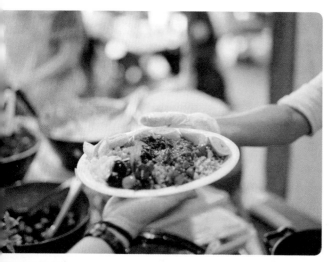

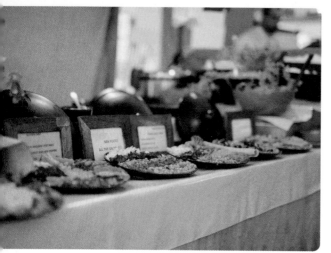

✤ ETHIOPIQUES 100% VEGAN

Long before veganism became a trend, there was Ethiopiques. Founder Elizabeth has been offering her healthy, plant-based food to market-goers of Brick Lane since 2006. With Ethiopian cuisine being naturally very accommodating to a vegan diet, Ethiopiques' dishes are based around pulses, grains and *injera* – the spongey, fermented flatbread used to scoop or mop up stews, curries and sauces. Try the set plate – mixing a little of everything – to try all the flavours in one sitting. The portions are large and can be made up of plant protein sources like chickpeas, lentils and soya beans, and the vegetables are plentiful. There's also a gluten-free plate and a three-sauce Injera Wrap. Elizabeth's food has gone from strength to strength, with a weekend stall at Southbank as well as Shoreditch – but her food is still as authentic and true to its roots as ever.

Market trader (check website for current locations)

www.instagram.com/ethiopiques

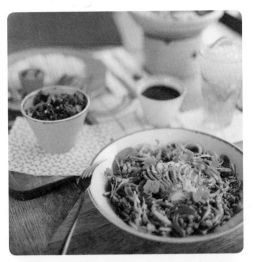

✤ LAS IGUANAS <u>VEGAN-FRIENDLY</u>

Bringing Latin American energy to London, Las Iguanas' five London restaurants will whisk you away to Central and South America through vibrant food, drink and decor. The vegetarian menu is packed with vegan options inspired by Mexican, Brazilian and Peruvian cuisine, and there's tapas as well as mains and unusual dessert options. Try the pan-fried Brazilian-style Palm Hearts to start, or go for the Holy Guacamole with spice-dusted corn chips. The Fiesta Ensalada is a solid option for a fresh and filling main – roasted butternut squash, avocado and oven-dried tomatoes are tossed in a poppy-seed dressing and placed on a bed of mixed leaves, topped with toasted seeds and charred corn. A creamy coconut pudding – the Tembleque, with mixed berries and a mango purée – will finish your flavour adventure on the sweetest note, and you'll be planning your next trip to Las Iguanas *enseguida*.

—

Peninsula Square, Millennium Way, SE10 0DX.
020 8312 8680
www.iguanas.co.uk
North Greenwich Tube.
Branches: Stratford E20 1ET, Wembley HA9 0FD,
plus two other locations across London.

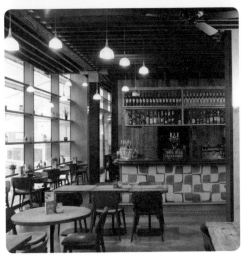

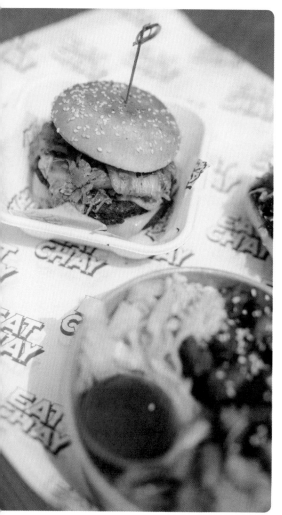

❖ EAT CHAY <u>100% VEGAN</u>

For London's best vegan Vietnamese food, follow Eat Chay from market to market as they serve up banh mi, buns and burgers inspired by childhood flavours with a vegan twist. *Chay* means 'vegan' in Vietnamese. Having grown their stall from humble beginnings at Brick Lane Market frying each piece of seitan with chopsticks, vegans and lovers of Vietnamese food now flock from all over London to try Eat Chay's plant-based creations; and there are also Korean-inspired options. The Chilli Lemongrass Bahn Mi Baguette is a must-try, with chilli lemongrass soya, a mushroom and walnut pâté, pickled carrots, coriander, cucumber and crispy onions, drizzled with sriracha mayo. Or go for the steamed bao buns – you get one fluffy steamed bun with Korean barbecue seitan, kimchi and sriracha mayo, and another with braised soya mince, pickled carrots and coriander, both filled with crispy onions. Eating *chay* never tasted so good.

—

48, Boxpark, 2–4 Bethnal Green Road, E1 6GY.
www.eatchay.com
Shoreditch High Street Overground.

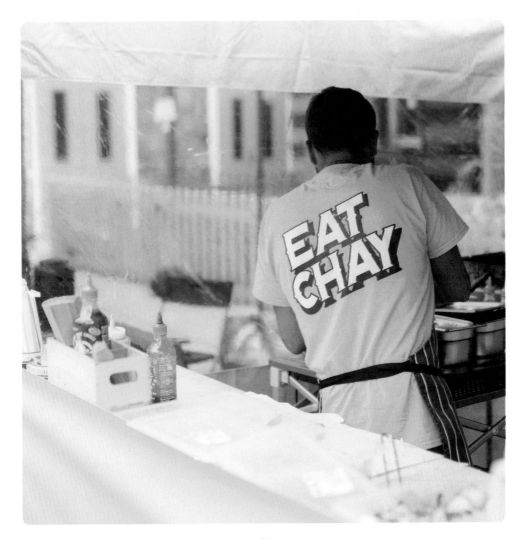

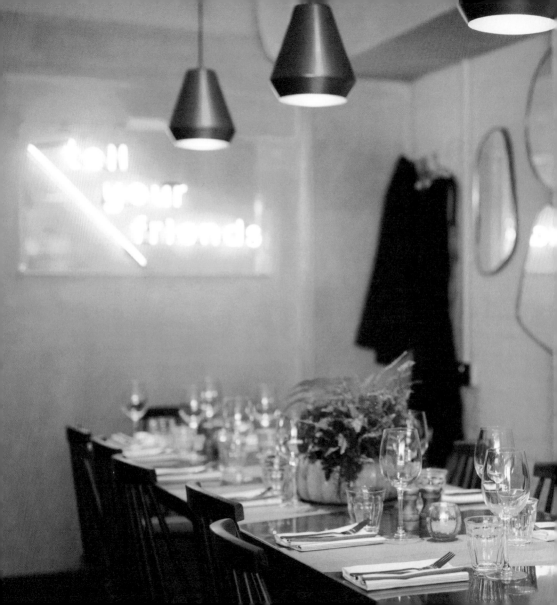

DATE NIGHT

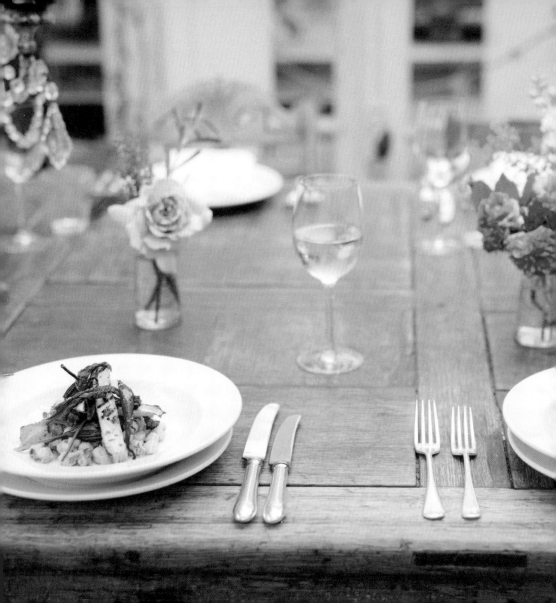

DATE NIGHT

Whether it's romantic ambience or a casual pub night you're after, London is quickly filling up with vegan-friendly places to wine and dine. Several pubs across town have recently had vegan makeovers, with seitan Sunday roasts and pub snacks proving popular with locals and vegans alike, while the fine-dining scene includes some of London's longest-standing vegan-friendly restaurants as well as some of the newest to open. With a mixture of places across north, east, south and west, you'll find an exciting itinerary no matter where you're headed.

Choose your restaurant and then plan your date – a West London wander ending with afternoon tea, a stroll through blossoming nurseries and a slice of chocolate cake – grab a friend or enjoy these experiences solo; the memories are waiting to be made.

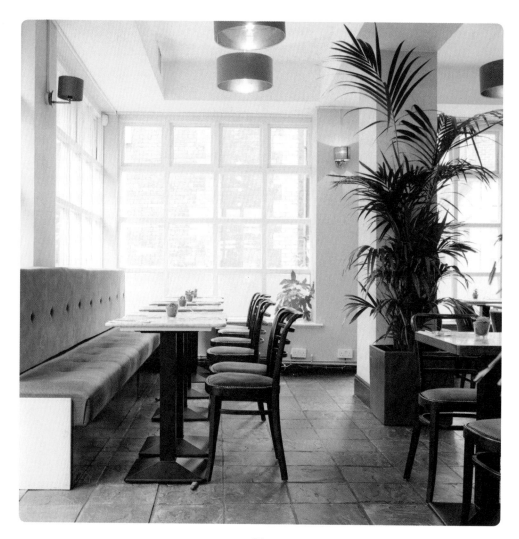

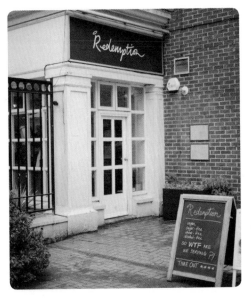

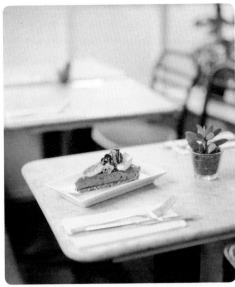

❖ REDEMPTION BAR 100% VEGAN

With a quick search for #redemptionbar on social media, you'll find scores of visitors posing with their angel-wing mural, boasting their 'redeemed' status after dining at London's most saintly restaurant. Redemption is proudly sober: a bar serving no alcohol, specialising in mocktails flavourful enough to rival the real thing. There are non-alcoholic takes on classics, such as the Pious Piña Colada, made with coconut kefir, and the Raspberry Royale with rose essence. If you're feeling more adventurous, go for the Activated Charcoal Martini topped with aquafaba.

As for the food, everything is vegan and wheat-free. Visit the easterly branch in Shoreditch or head west to Covent Garden or Notting Hill – at each branch, you'll find guilt-free plant-based food and spoil yourself, as the Redemption motto goes, without spoiling yourself.

—

320 Old Street, EC1V 9DR.
020 7613 0720
www.redemptionbar.co.uk
Old Street Tube.
Branches: Notting Hill W2 5BH, Covent Garden WC2H 9AT.

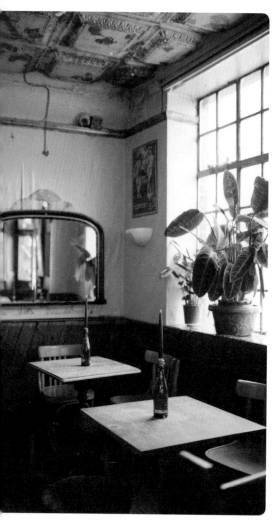

✤ THE DOVE VEGAN-FRIENDLY

At the heart of bustling Broadway Market lies The Dove, a Belgian pub whose vegan offerings are surprisingly plentiful. With the aim to have half their menu meat-free, there are vegan starters, mains and desserts to enjoy, and there's even a Sunday roast dinner with all the trimmings. Weekday mains include a nori-wrapped tofu 'fish' and chips, with the tofu battered in a Belgian beer coating, and a Thai Massaman Pie – a mild coconutty curry pie with seitan chunks and sweet potato, created by their talented Thai chef. And if you'd prefer a burger, try the Pea and Black Sesame Burger with black olives and rosemary, served with vegan wasabi mayonnaise and pickle, or the Nut Roast Burger with pistachio and flaked almonds. A pint of sweet-potato or regular fries complements the burgers perfectly.

24/28 Broadway Market, E8 4QJ.
020 7275 7617
www.dovepubs.com
Cambridge Heath Overground.

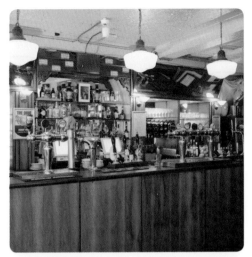

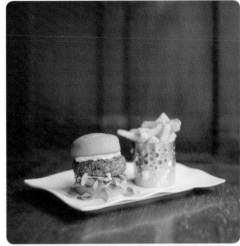

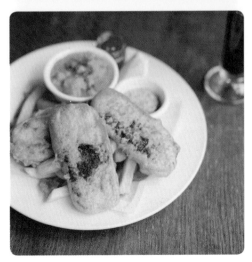

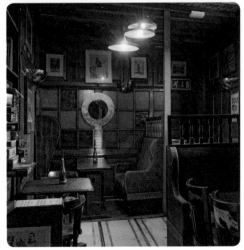

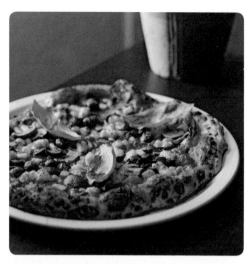

✦ FED BY WATER 100% VEGAN

FED By Water starts with a simple idea. Water is the life source of everything, and the purer the water, the tastier and healthier the food. FED By Water is a gourmet Italian restaurant that strives to replicate fine Italian cuisine, but without meat or dairy. They're passionate about plant-based food, serving an exclusively vegan menu. This passion extends to their starters and desserts, with their in-house team making everything from their own cheese platters to their excessively decadent chocolate pizza. FED By Water serve a mean seitan carbonara and they don't scrimp on the serving sizes either. If Nonna was vegan, this is what she'd serve you each Sunday – or a thick wedge of FED's lasagna. While FED might not have the rustic Italian charm of a downtown trattoria, it's clear that their food validates FED's status as one of London's best vegan Italian restaurants.

———

59 Kingsland High Street, E8 2JS.

07490 637 200

www.fedbywater.co.uk

Dalston Kingsland Overground.

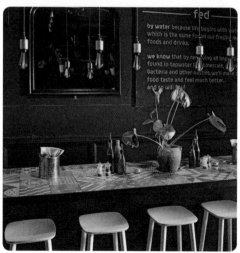

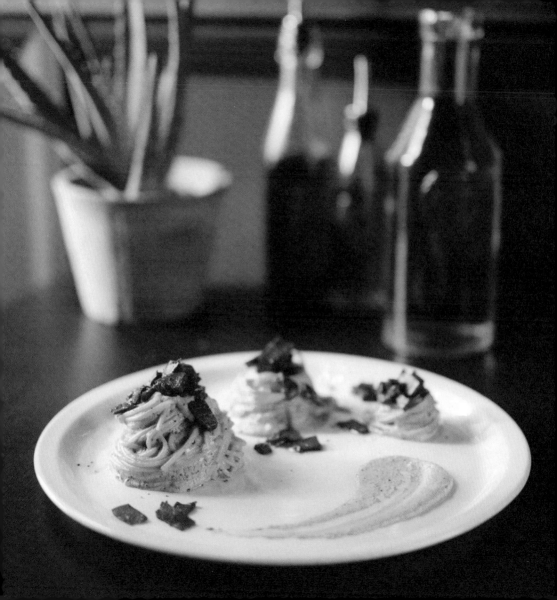

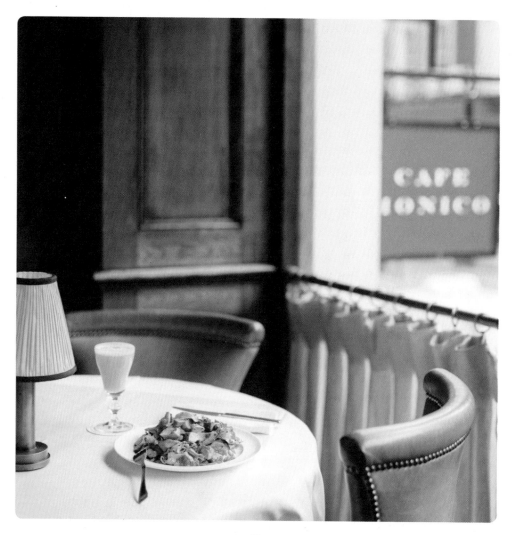

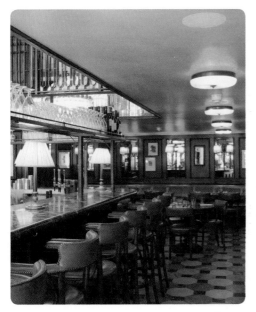

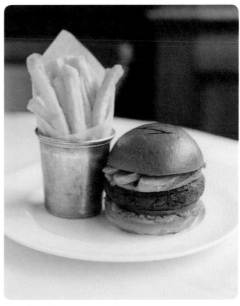

✤ CAFE MONICO VEGAN-FRIENDLY

Brasseries are often less accommodating to vegan diets, but Cafe Monico is proud in offering continental plant-based dishes to the exquisite standard you'd expect from a Soho House restaurant. Resurrected from its original site nearby, which opened in 1877 and closed to make way for the expanding Piccadilly Circus in the 1950s, Cafe Monico is now situated close to the Apollo and Palace theatres. There are always vegan options on their seasonal menu, such as the Aubergine Mazzetta Spaghetti and the Stuffed Aubergine with tomato and pesto – the vegan dishes are labelled clearly too. For a more leafy lunch, opt for one of Cafe Monico's classic salads – their Butter Lettuce and Avocado Salad allows for creamy indulgence while remaining a light and fresh dish, satisfying meat-eaters and vegans alike. And for dessert, try one of the zingy sorbets.

—

39–45 Shaftesbury Avenue, W1D 6LA.
020 3727 6161
www.cafemonico.com
Piccadilly Circus Tube.

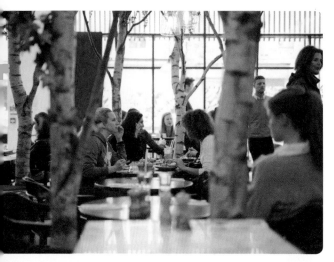

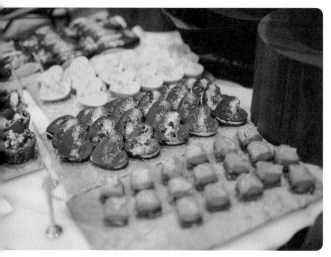

❖ ETHOS VEGAN-FRIENDLY

Take a break from shopping on Oxford
Street to refuel with unprocessed,
innovative food from Ethos, situated
just a minute's walk from the high
street. You'll find vegetarian dishes
from all around the world with about
50 percent of dishes suitable for vegans
and, with the pay-by-weight concept,
you can happily try a bit of everything.
All of Ethos's food is made from scratch
each day, with ingredients locally
sourced where possible, and there's no
microwave in their kitchen. If you're
looking for a healthier special-occasion
experience, Ethos offer a plant-based
afternoon tea. The changing menu
features dishes such as broccoli and
beetroot muffins, plus blueberry scones
with cashew cream. To drink, there's
a large selection of finest-quality teas,
including a rhubarb and vanilla Chinese
green tea and an herbal rooibos blend
flavoured with marzipan.

48 Eastcastle Street, W1W 8DX.
020 3581 1538
www.ethosfoods.com
Oxford Street Tube.

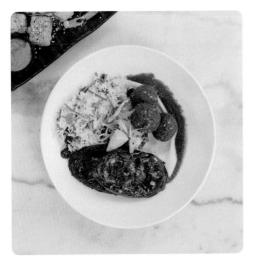

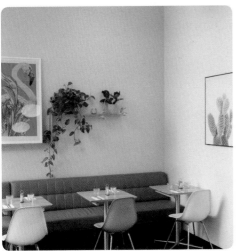

✤ MILDREDS <u>VEGAN-FRIENDLY</u>

One of London's best-known vegetarian restaurants, Mildreds has been a top pick for birthday celebrations, romantic dates and work meetings ever since the original Soho restaurant opened in 1988. Each branch has its own unique personality – head to Lexington Street for a cosy family meal; or for brunch in an industrial-chic setting bursting with natural light, head to Pentonville Road in King's Cross for blueberry quinoa and oat waffles with coconut cream. When London vegans think of Mildreds, the dishes that spring to mind are the vegetable gyoza starter, the Polish Burger – with beetroot, white bean, basil mayo and pickled cabbage in a brioche bun – and the peanut-butter brownie with vegan ice cream. Mildreds don't take bookings, so visiting at off-peak times will help you get a table faster – even with a queue, it's well worth the wait.

—

1 Dalston Square, Dalston Lane, E8 3GU.
020 8017 1815
www.mildreds.co.uk
Dalston Junction or.Dalston Kingland Overground
Branches: Soho W1F 9AN, King's Cross N1 9JP,
plus one other location in Camden.

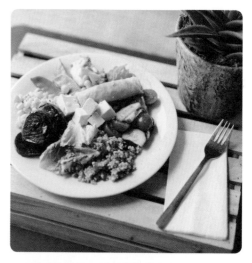

✤ TIBITS VEGAN-FRIENDLY

Tibits is truly for all occasions and appetites. With a large food boat of exclusively vegetarian options and plenty of vegan fare to choose from, the pay-by-weight approach allows diners to enjoy exactly what they fancy: no more, no less. There are both hot and cold dishes, breads, salads and a range of desserts. The buffet changes seasonally, but you can expect to enjoy some of the more regular options such as the curry and coconut udon, vegetable tartar and the infamous and ever-present sticky toffee pudding (it's too good not to have all year round). Both the Heddon Street and the Bankside branches are great destinations for brunch, lunch or dinner – and the quality of the drinks menu matches the food. For something different, try the cashew jambo made with homemade cashew milk, coconut milk, dates and garam masala.

12–14 Heddon Street, W1B 4DA.

020 7758 4112

www.tibits.co.uk

Oxford Circus or Piccadilly Circus Tube.

Branches: Bankside SE1 0SW.

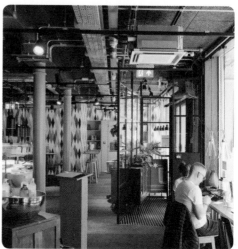

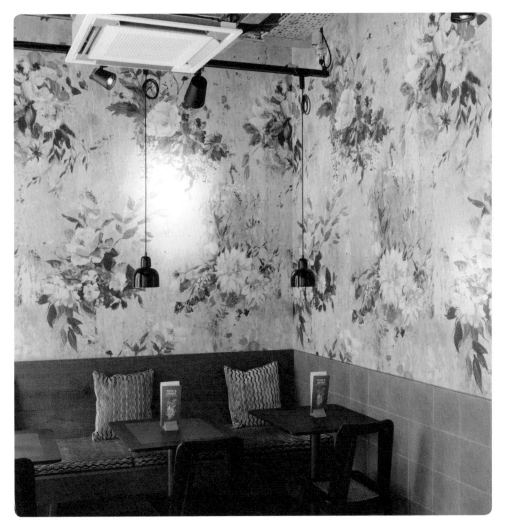

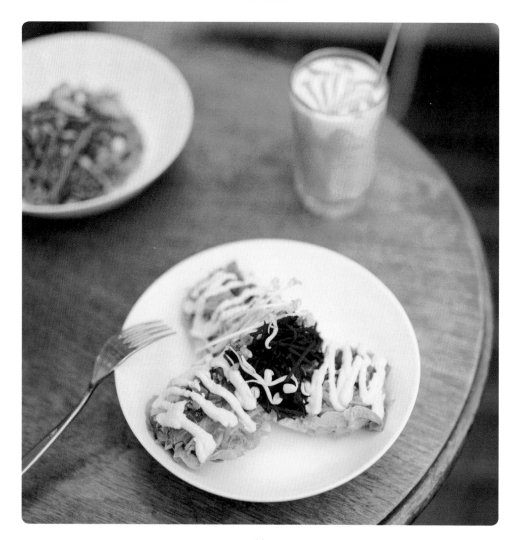

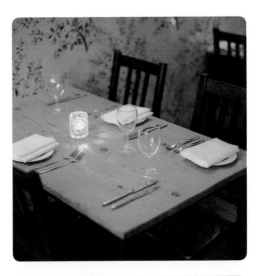

❖ MANNA <u>100% VEGAN</u>

The leafy, residential area of Primrose Hill plays host to Manna, one of Europe's oldest vegetarian establishments spanning over 50 years. Manna is known for its traditional vegan Sunday roast – a staple on their menu for the past ten years. Manna is fully committed to serving a plant-based menu with a range of organic vegan wine, as well as a selection of vegan cakes from their own certified bakery. Making the most of their location, Manna also offers a picnic hamper, which provides treats and snacks for up to six people, taken either from their full menu or one of their daily specials – perfect for a walk along the nearby canal or a picnic on Primrose Hill. Manna is an ideal stopover when exploring Camden, London Zoo or Regent's Canal and offers classic food with a vegan twist, boasting an eclectic menu from burgers and fries to bangers and mash.

----

4 Erskine Road, Primrose Hill, NW3 3AJ.
020 7722 8028
www.mannav.com
Chalk Farm Tube.

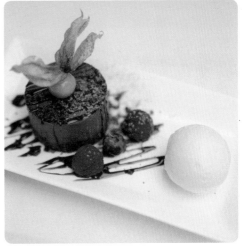

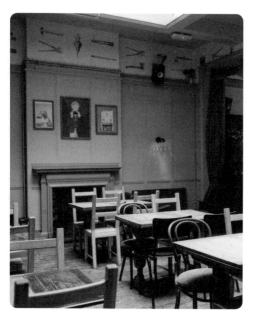

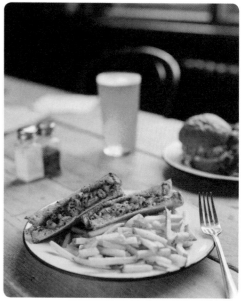

✤ THE BLACKSMITH
& THE TOFFEEMAKER 100% VEGAN

If you're on the hunt for an ethical pub, The Blacksmith & The Toffeemaker have you covered. Holding the belief that omitting meat and dairy from the menu makes for a more sustainable establishment, the entire menu is vegan, while still offering precisely the kind of dishes you'd expect at a pub. There's the Aloo Tikka Burger, championing the UK's love of Indian-British fusion cuisine, the vegan Halloumi and Kimchi Burger with pickles, burger sauce and shredded lettuce, and for afters

there's a bread and butter pudding made with banana, cinnamon and dates. Going one step further on the sustainability front, The Blacksmith & The Toffeemaker send the majority of their bar waste to recycling, and their food waste is used to create renewable energy through anaerobic digestion. So the next time you fancy a pub quiz on a Monday night, you know where to go.

—

292–294 St John Street, EC1V 4PA.
www.theblacksmithandthetoffeemaker.co.uk
Angel or Farringdon Tube.

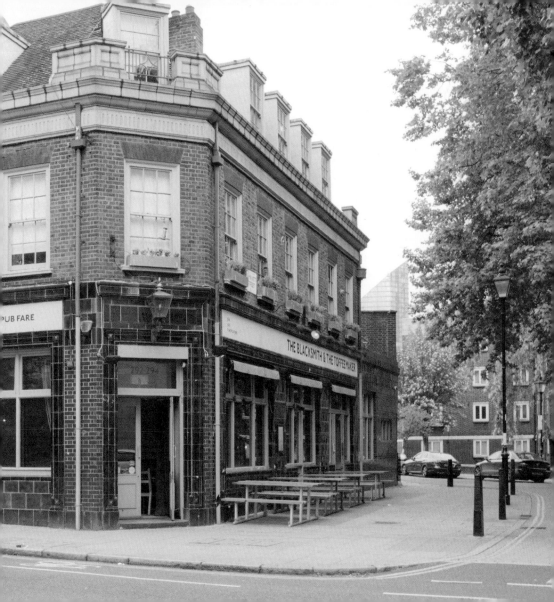

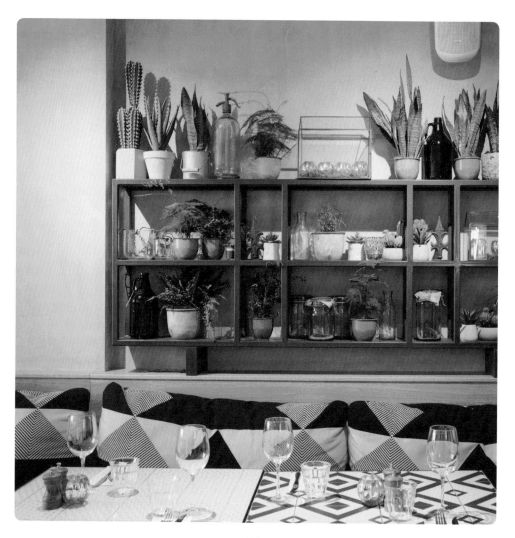

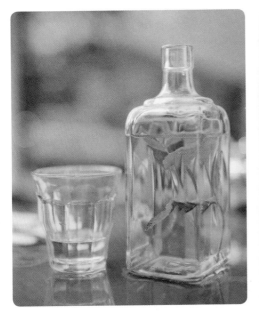

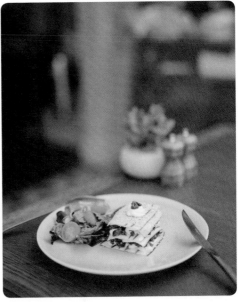

✤ TELL YOUR FRIENDS 100% VEGAN

Have you ever eaten breaded banana blossom in a restaurant? Probably not. Paired with a cashew tartare sauce, Tell Your Friends' take on a vegan fish and chips dish is welcomingly creative in a city filling fast with samey vegan options as the movement continues to grow. On TYF's menu, comfort food favourites like this are nestled among refreshing options such as the Japanese Raw Bowl with cauliflower rice and daikon, and the Buddha Bowl with sticky tofu, pak choi and a sweet sesame sauce. Founded by Lucy and Tiffany Watson, the vegan sisters are using their fame for good by promoting cruelty-free dining to their non-vegan fans as well as providing a great new spot for vegans. The interior at Tell Your Friends is as fresh and beautiful as the food itself, with pretty glassware and indoor plants bringing the atmosphere alive.

175 New King's Road, SW6 4SW.
020 7731 6404
www.tellyourfriendsldn.com
Parsons Green Tube.

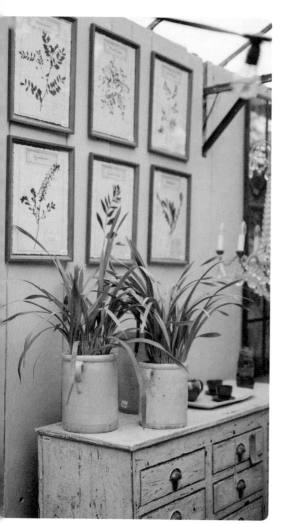

✤ **PETERSHAM NURSERIES** VEGAN-FRIENDLY

Although Petersham Nurseries is so much more than a restaurant, it shouldn't be overlooked as one of London's best places to eat. Cakes, sandwiches, salads and hot dishes are served in an elegant wooden teahouse, with the food's English and Italian themes reflecting the locally sourced seasonal ingredients. For no-nonsense indulgence, their chocolate cake is not to be missed. The flexibility of a lighter, more casual meal in the greenhouse-turned-teahouse and the more formal approach of the restaurant makes Petersham Nurseries a delightful establishment for any occasion, and is always worth a visit when in the area (there's now a more urban branch in Covent Garden too). It's never a bad thing when you can pop in for lunch and head home with a scented candle and a new houseplant to add to the collection.

—

Church Lane, Off Petersham Road, Richmond, TW10 7AB.
020 8940 5230
www.petershamnurseries.com
Richmond Tube (25 minute walk).
Branches: Covent Garden WC2E 9FB.

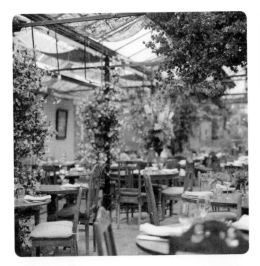

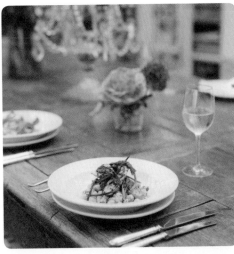

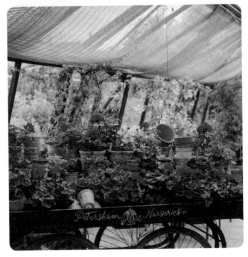

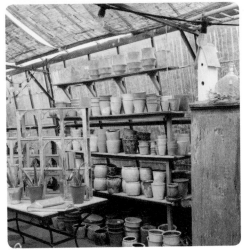

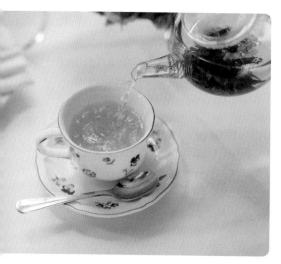

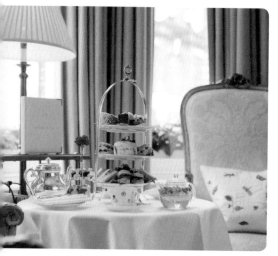

❧ EGERTON HOUSE HOTEL <u>VEGAN-FRIENDLY</u>

This historic, 5-star hotel in the heart of London's most affluent area – Knightsbridge – offers one of the best vegan afternoon teas in the capital. A stone's throw away from the V&A museum, the hotel oozes prestige and is a real treat for visitors looking for a true English dining experience. Their vegan afternoon tea, provided with excellent service, comes with a range of fine teas, a selection of delightful cakes – chocolate, vanilla and custard flavoured – and small, bite-sized sandwiches. Fillings and toppings include grilled veggies, guacamole, olive tapenade and of course the simple but traditional slice of cucumber. The Egerton House Hotel is a perfect stopover when exploring the museum district of West London and is a great representation of classical British food culture. You won't be out of place here sipping your tea with your pinkie in the air.

17–19 Egerton Terrace, Knightsbridge, SW3 2BX.
020 7589 2412
www.egertonhousehotel.com
South Kensington Tube.

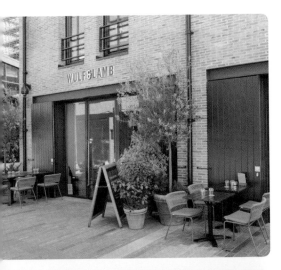

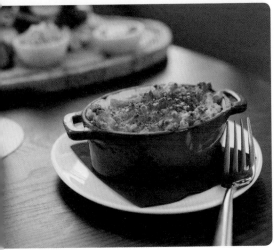

❖ WULF & LAMB 100% VEGAN

Voted 'Most Loved Local Restaurant in Chelsea' in *Time Out's* Love London Awards 2018, Wulf & Lamb's menu has everything you fancy, from nutrient-packed salads to creamy linguine. With marble tables and great natural light setting the mood perfectly for a modern vegan dining experience, this is a great restaurant for brunch with friends or to indulge in some vegan 'wine time'. For breakfast, it has to be the Full Wulf: a potato layer cake with borlotti bean ragoût, scrambled ackee, lemony spinach and sautéed peppers with toasted sourdough. Most-loved lunch and dinner options include the Cashew Mac 'n' Cheese (crunchy on the outside, creamy underneath) and the Green Coconut Curry with sweet potato mash and jasmine rice. End with a Mango and Passion Fruit Cheesecake, topped with raspberry crumble and mint, and leave Wulf & Lamb a happy herbivore.

—

243 Pavilion Road, SW1X 0BP.
020 3948 5999
www.wulfandlamb.com
Sloane Square Tube.

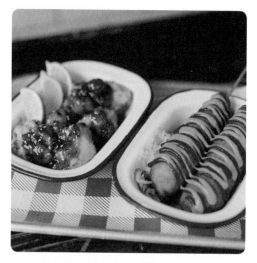

✤ THE FULL NELSON <u>VEGAN-FRIENDLY</u>

There are dog-friendly restaurants, and then
there are restaurants that really love dogs, and
a scroll through The Full Nelson's Instagram
page will tell you which group the bar falls
into – so animal lovers can expect a double thrill
in Deptford, combining furry company and a
vegan meal for a memorable lunch experience.
As for the food, The Full Nelson proudly offers
indulgent vegan junk food, from a range of
burgers through to their Seitanic Wings.
The Colonel burger is an obvious choice: crispy
coated 'chicken' with a garlic buffalo sauce.
Or try the Dogwood Corn Dogs, dipped in a corn
batter with mustard, sauerkraut and pickles.
The menu is completely vegetarian, and all
menu items can be made vegan – so expect
your dog-walking route to detour to Deptford
Broadway regularly from now on.

—

47 Deptford Broadway, SE8 4PH.
www.thefullnelsondeptford.co.uk
Deptford Bridge DLR.

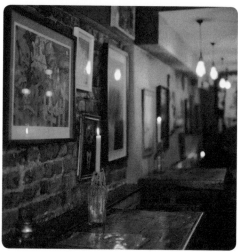

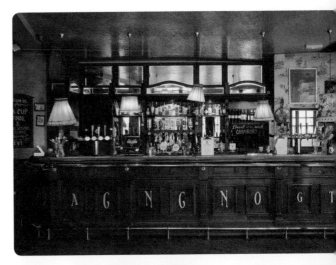

✤ THE TIGER <u>VEGAN-FRIENDLY</u>

An 'omni' pub that's 'herbi'-friendly, The Tiger splits its food menu down the middle – with the omnivorous options on one side and the vegetarian options on the other – and encourages diners to eat with their hands and not take life too seriously. Chow down on street-food-inspired fare while sampling local and regional real ales or opt for a craft beer instead. Among the classic pub food is the Not Hog – a seitan sausage with ketchup and French fries, and a 'classic bun' with vegan cheddar and relish. As well as weekday bites, mains and sides, The Tiger showcases all that's good about hearty vegan comfort food with both of their 'herbi' Sunday roast options being suitable for vegans: there's a choice of Seitan Joint and Chestnut Mushroom Nut Roast, both accompanied by vegan Yorkshire puddings on request. Come for a drink, stay for the food.

---

18 Camberwell Green, SE5 7AA.
020 7703 5246
www.thetigerpub.com
Denmark Hill Overground.

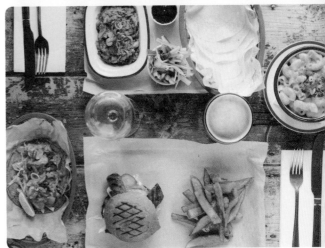

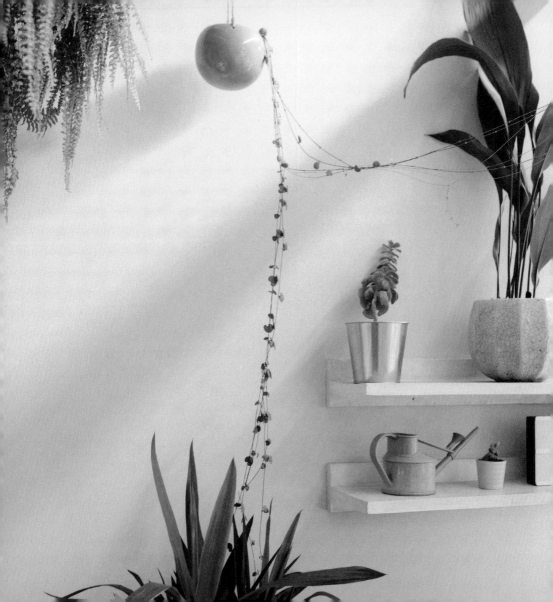

PLANT POWER

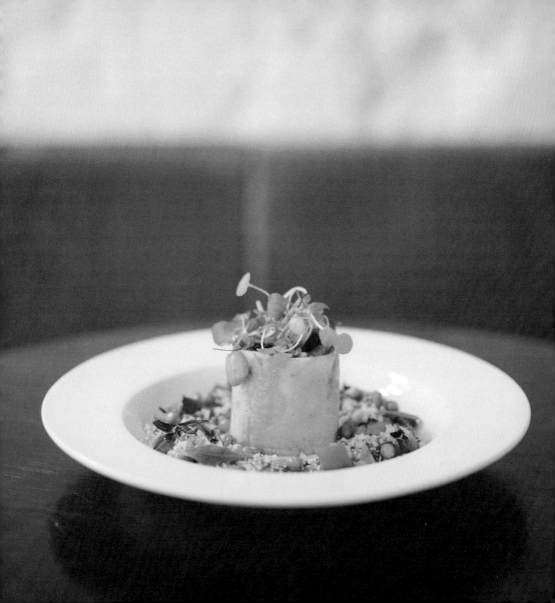

PLANT POWER

Bacon made from smoky coconut shavings, caramel made from medjool dates, pizza bases made from dried seeds and tomato – the creativity of plant-based chefs is something to be admired. Carefully crafting nutrient-rich alternatives to junk food while championing loaded rainbow-coloured salads and proving that plants contain protein, too, the plant-powered vegans of London are real movers and shakers, and their growing audience spans a huge free-from demographic as well as fellow vegans. If you're dairy-free, gluten-free or even soy-free, a lot of these establishments will be able to cater for you without foregoing flavour, and are slowly convincing diners to eat the same way every day with their filling meals leaving bellies full but not stuffed. Plant power feels good because it's all good, so be ready for these eateries to tempt you to the bright side.

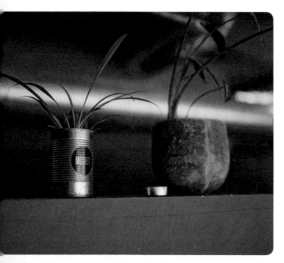

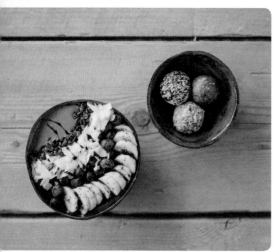

✤ MOTHER <u>100% VEGAN</u>

Family-owned juice bar MOTHER sits just off Regent's Canal and is the perfect pit-stop after a morning jog by the water. Stepping inside, you'll see as many plants as you did on your jog – decorating the interior as well as on your plate. It's a green haven contrasting with the industrial backdrop of Hackney Wick, and a real breath of fresh air for East London. Open for breakfast, lunch and dinner, their food spans everything from loaded acai bowls to sausage rolls and pulled jackfruit and bean chilli. Their focus is on local and organic produce, with juices made onsite daily and a frequently changing menu. All juices are raw, cold-pressed and have a high vegetable content, making them some of the highest-quality juices you'll find in London. Expect to see regulars working from here, dog in tow and sipping home-brewed kombucha or oat milk coffee.

———

1, Canalside, Here East Estate, E20 3BS.
07388 554 060
www.mother.works
Hackney Wick Overground.

✤ MOOSHIES 100% VEGAN

Junk food, but not as you know it. Mooshies takes
all the fast-food classics – burgers, fries, deep-fried
cheese sticks and milkshakes – and turns them
into vegan cheat day treats by using plant-based
ingredients. The Fillet-Om-Phish burger, for
example, is made from battered aubergine and
nori – a genius combination of texture and flavour
creating a burger that's indulgent and satisfying.
Founders John and Nelly have created a venue
that feels laid-back and relaxed even on a Saturday
night when the restaurant is full. They've brought
Shoreditch inside, with street art on the walls
giving the place a real punch of character that's
missing from a lot of the carbon-copy restaurants
up and down Brick Lane, and their food is equally
as intriguing – who would have thought that
pulled barbecue jackfruit would make a convincing
replacement for pulled pork?

—

104 Brick Lane, E1 6RL.
07931 842 458
www.veganburger.org
Aldgate East Tube or Shoreditch High Street Overground.

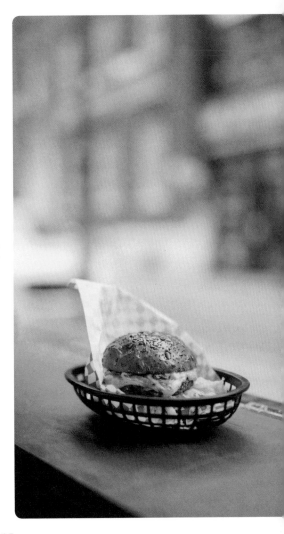

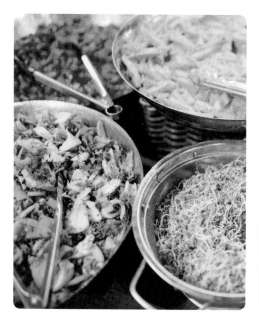

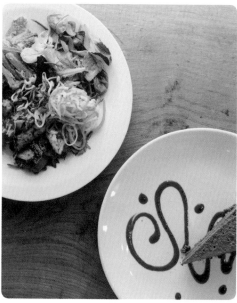

☘ VANTRA LOUNGEVITY <u>100% VEGAN</u>

If you've ever been to Bali, you won't be able to help comparing the peaceful, sanctuary vibe of its yogi-enticing health-food cafés to Soho's Vantra. It feels spiritual, high-quality and unpretentious all at once, and you get the feeling that the restaurant's very walls are looking out for your wellbeing. Vantra opened in 1999 and has since become a favourite among both seasoned vegans and newbies with its natural, all-vegan raw and steamed cuisine. With a truly inclusive approach to food, the restaurant caters to a huge array of diets, including kosher, halal and low-sugar as well as plant-based. Choose from a healthful buffet of delicious dishes like mushroom stroganoff or lentil stew, with sides such as Raw Cucumber Kimchi (fermented with probiotics). Follow with a raw cake and a superfood cocktail, either non-alcoholic or alcoholic – they're open till 11pm.

—

5 Wardour Street, W1D 6PB.
020 7287 5222
www.vantra.co.uk
Piccadilly Circus Tube, Leicester Square Tube.

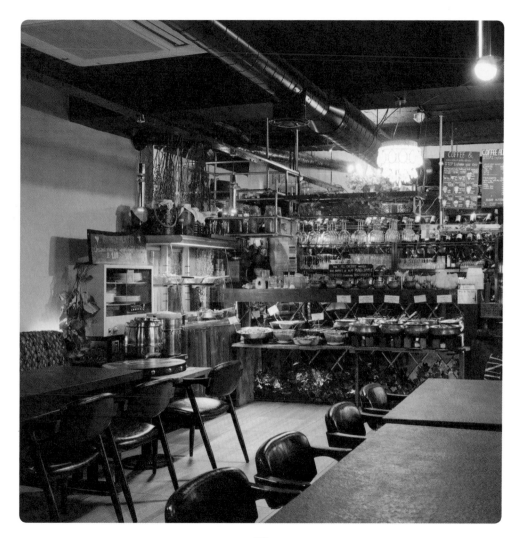

✤ OSU COCONUTS 100% VEGAN

Head to Brick Lane Market on a Sunday and you'll find Benny slicing open coconuts with a machete. Londoners can enjoy hot coconut 'tea' or fresh cold coconut water straight from the source, along with Benny's famous pancakes. With a young green coconut base that's naturally gluten-free, there are sweet options including apple cinnamon crumble, plus savoury options like the Aunt Patricia – a plantain fritter base with mango, a pumpkin roti mix and Caribbean coleslaw – inspired by Benny's aunt's Jamaican-Indian cooking. This is creative plant-based food at its finest, priced affordably and made with passion. Find these pancakes in Shoreditch, Camden and Broadway Market – check online for locations and days. OSU also run OSU Lifestyle, a charitable clothing line funded by OSU Coconuts, with 100 percent of profits going to children or adults suffering from illness. Supporting this small business feels good and does good.

—

Market trader
(check website for current location)
www.osucoconuts.com

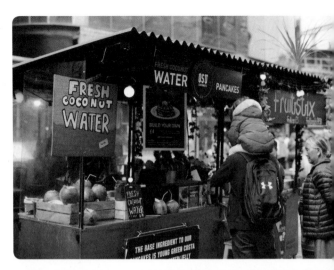

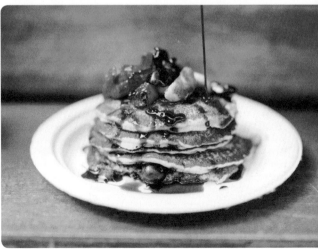

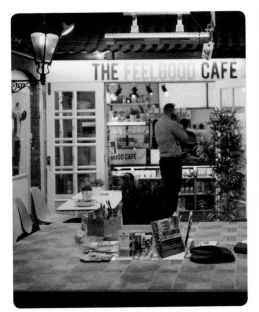

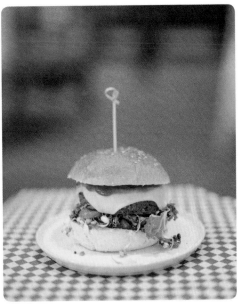

✤ THE FEEL GOOD CAFÉ 100% VEGAN

If every Station Road in London was home to a Feel Good Café, the city would be a better, healthier place. Vegan food evangelists Idan and Izabela have brought a world of plant-based goodness to unsuspecting Chingford through a tasty menu of breakfast and lunch foods. For lunch, try their Stew of the Day with lentils or beans, basmati rice and changing vegetables, and either warm up with the Liquid Bounty Hot Chocolate or cool down with their cold blend of double espresso, almond milk, maple syrup and vegan ice cream. And there's a great opportunity for those with green fingers who want to help diners eat organically grown vegetables: ask the team about The Feel Good Café's volunteering scheme, where you can help out at their nearby Pimp Hall allotment site in exchange for meals and drinks at the café.

The Village Arcade, 49 Station Road, E4 7DA.
07799 965 611
www.thefeelgoodcafe.com
Chingford Overground.

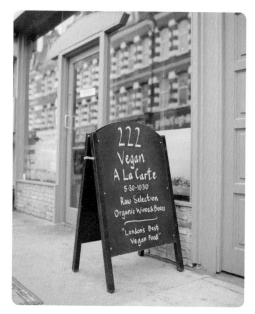

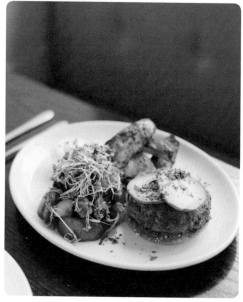

♣ 222 VEGAN CUISINE 100% VEGAN

An evening spent at 222 Vegan Cuisine is a real treat for the body and soul: get fed nourishing, natural foods while keeping the indulgence at chocolate-gateau level. With a menu designed by internationally renowned chef Ben Asamani, your appetite and your curiosity will be well looked after at 222 as the creativity flows through dishes like the oyster mushroom and spinach raclette with a tofu cottage cheese, and the Medallions and Mash consisting of seitan medallions, potato and parsnip mash and an onion gravy. If you had the warm chocolate gateau for dessert on your last visit, it might be time for the Spice Island Pie with raw cashew cream on a crunchy base. Finish your visit to North End Road by heading to GreenBay, London's first vegan supermarket, just a stone's throw away from the restaurant.

222 North End Road, W14 9NU.
020 7381 2322
www.222vegan.com
West Kensington Tube or West Brompton Overground.

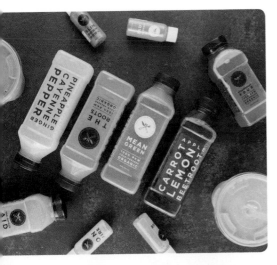

✤ JUICEBABY 100% VEGAN

Taking the juice bar concept to Kensington levels, Juicebaby use only the best ingredients to provide nutrient-powerhouse salads with mix and match dressings in a beautifully clean, contemporary setting – they've recently opened a second branch in Notting Hill too. In Juicebaby's fridges, you'll find big bottles of nut milks produced in small batches and blended with flavours like vanilla and coffee, to be enjoyed with their caramel bars made from coconut, cashews, macadamia nuts, maple syrup and raw chocolate. Their juices are never watered down or pasteurised, and they never add sugar to them either. Expect to enjoy your meal alongside groups of yogis dropping in after class as well as regulars with their dogs. With a philosophy of switching unhealthier foods for more wholesome ones little by little, Juicebaby are helping turn West London vegan one açai bowl at a time.

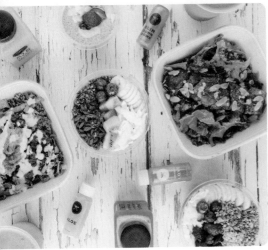

398 Kings Road, SW10 0LJ.
020 7351 2230
www.juicebaby.co.uk
South Kensington or Fulham Broadway Tube.
Branches: Notting Hill W11 2SB.

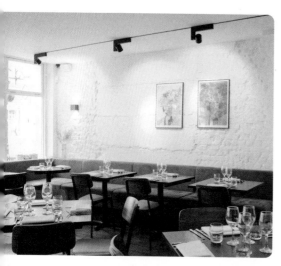

❖ THE GATE VEGAN-FRIENDLY

If you're after an afternoon of al fresco dining complete with wine, The Gate is West London's most obvious choice. Many new vegans are unaware that wine is sometimes produced using fining agents made from animal products, and this often goes unlabelled, so it's refreshing when a restaurant serves only vegan-friendly wines. These are a speciality at The Gate, with a great natural wine list to work your way through on their beautiful Hammersmith garden terrace or in their outdoor seating at the Marylebone branch. And if the weather doesn't lend itself to an outdoor meal, the cosmopolitan yet ambient setting at all four of The Gate's locations will have time pass you by while enjoying menu favourites such as Miso-glazed Aubergine, Mushroom Rotolo and their famous chunky herb polenta chips.

—

51A Queen Caroline Street, Hammersmith, W6 9QL.
020 8748 6932
www.thegaterestaurants.com
Hammersmith Tube.
Branches: Marylebone W1H 7NL, Islington EC1V 4NN,
St John's Wood NW8 7AS.

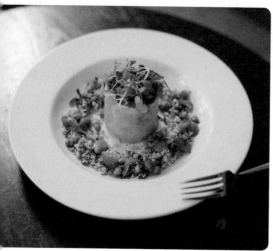

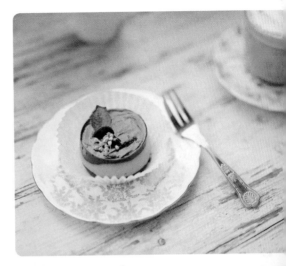

❧ PARADISE PLANTBASED <u>100% VEGAN</u>

Healthy never looked this good. Since graduating
from raw-food stall to full café in 2016, Paradise
Plantbased has become one of West London's
favourite plant-based food destinations –
attracting vegans with the food, and non-vegans
with the aesthetic (who'll come back when they
discover just how good the food is). Choose from
a generous menu, with plenty of raw and gluten-
free options – for breakfast, try the chickpea
omelette with mashed avocado and an 'eggy'
cashew sauce, and for lunch, go for the signature
Raw Paradise Pizza with a tomato and sunseed
base, cashew cheese and a fragrant pesto. There's
also a selection of desserts from founder and
chef, Egle, that is 'free from all the bad stuff and
full of goodness'. Paradise Plantbased sets the bar
high with its interior, but it's the food and drink
that really take the (raw) cake.

---

59 Chamberlayne Road, NW10 3ND.
020 8968 8321
www.paradiseplantbased.com
Kensal Rise Overground or Kensal Green Tube.

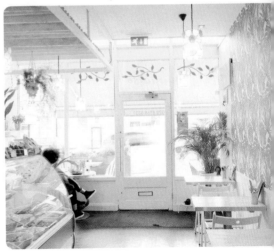

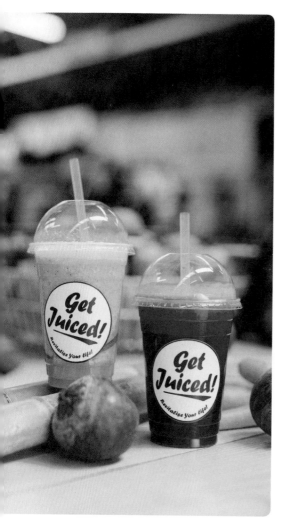

✤ GET JUICED 100% VEGAN

Get Juiced is home to some of London's most colourful and healthful food. The menu boasts organic, cold-pressed juices, salads, cakes, acai bowls, sugar-cane juice and more, and they also offer juice cleanses. The eatery is located at Tooting Market where you can enjoy juices like founder Leon's favourite, Jack the Lad, made with jackfruit, avocado, lime, apple, mango and orange and the Pineapple Punch with organic Ghanaian pineapple, coconut milk, almonds, Irish moss, dates, CBD oil and vanilla. After your juice, feast on specials to the tune of raw vegan patties stuffed with spinach, sun-dried tomatoes and olives, laced with Scotch bonnet, and smashed avocado on top of spiced coconut pancakes. Be sure to rack the brains of Leon and the team about the nutritional benefits of the food and drink they offer – they're a passionate, knowledgeable and healthy bunch.

Tooting Market, Unit 15A, 21–23 Tooting High Street, SW17 0SN

07857 803 781

www.facebook.com/getjuicedbar

Tooting Broadway Tube.

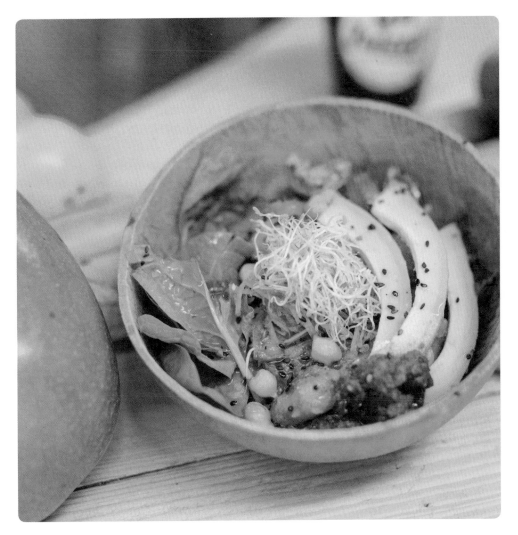

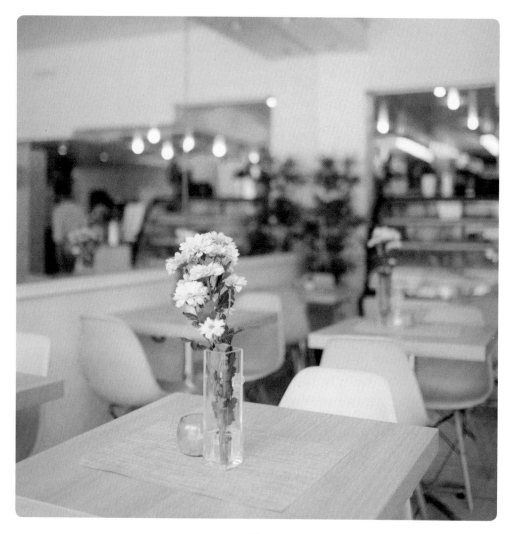

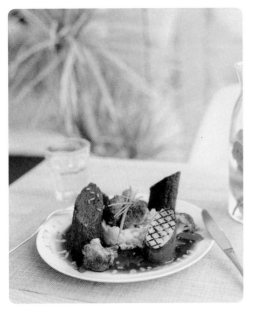
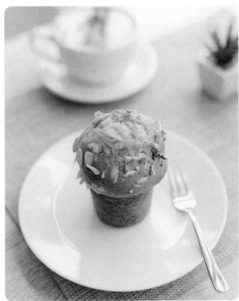

✤ VEGAN EXPRESS 100% VEGAN

When Vegan Express founders Charles and Ulrika went through their own lifestyle change in 2013, they decided to draw on Charles' two decades of culinary experience – including years at The Dorchester – to open a restaurant with a mission to make vegan mainstream. Tooting is now home to this wonderfully light and airy venue, where vegans and non-vegans alike can enjoy healthy bean burgers, sweet and savoury waffles, sticky toffee pudding and more. The drinks menu spans an array of vegan wines, pale ale and kombucha, and their hot drinks can be made with a choice of soya, rice, coconut or almond milk. On top of excluding animal products from their menu, the Vegan Express team are focused on sourcing food locally and keeping their food's environmental footprint as low as possible. Eat here knowing you're enjoying some of London's most ethically sound food.

—

913 Garratt Lane, SW17 0LT.
020 8127 6560
www.veganexpress.co.uk
Tooting Broadway Tube.

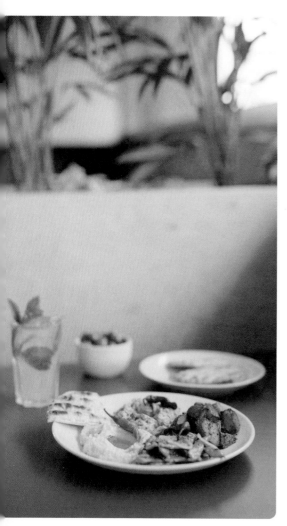

✤ WILDFLOWER VEGAN-FRIENDLY

Wildflower by name, wildflower by nature – adding a flash of greenery to the converted car park that is Peckham Levels, this jungalow-vibe vegetarian and vegan canteen serves pastries and cakes, lunch, dinner and there's brunch on the weekends. Wildflower's menu changes daily, but cakes are among the likes of vegan banana bread and chocolate brownie; lunch can range from panzanella to hummus and flatbread (there's a kids' plate of this too); and for brunch you might find their vegan Full English or their harissa-scrambled tofu with wild garlic on sourdough toast. For those spoilt for choice, try the Sampling Menu, of which there's a fully vegan version. And if you're looking for a meal with a view, Wildflower is a great choice – head to Rye Lane and see for yourself.

Peckham Levels, 95A Rye Lane, SE15 4ST.
020 3735 3775
www.wildflowerpeckham.uk
Peckham Rye Overground.

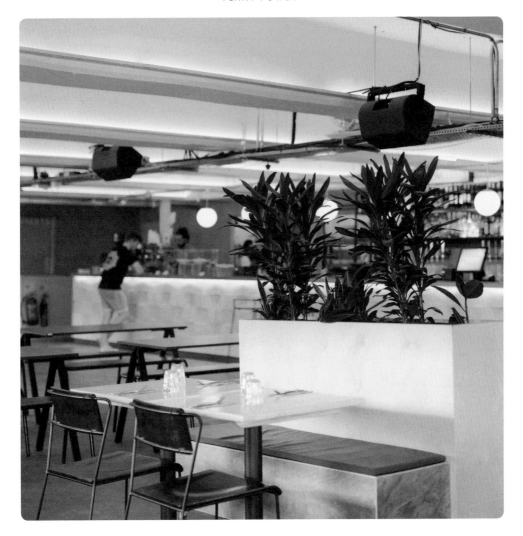

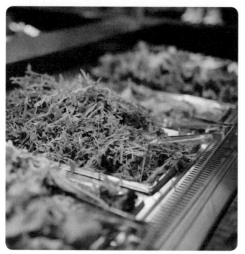

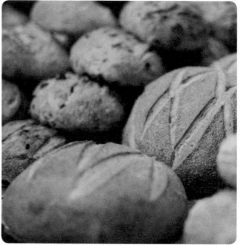

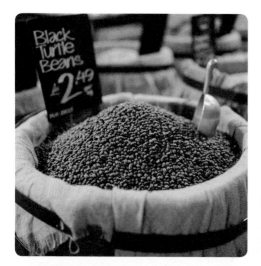

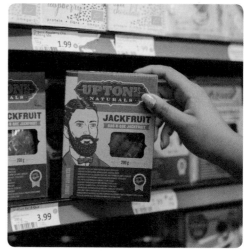

✤ WHOLE FOODS MARKET VEGAN-FRIENDLY

While Whole Foods is famous across the US and the UK for its abundant selection of vegan products, the larger stores are also the ideal place to go if you're looking for free-from food to eat in or take away. Although not a fully vegan supermarket, Whole Foods specialise in providing the finest selection of vegan brands, encompassing fresh and prepared food, drinks and even supplements. The flagship store in Kensington has a whole floor dedicated to eating in. Here, find a plethora of freshly made vegan options, including burritos and crispy edible bowls filled with beans, rice, veg and sauce. The freshest refrigerated food can also be found across stores, with treats like tofu cheesecake and spinach tortillas ready to go – bring your reusable cutlery (to be extra eco-friendly) and watch the crowds go by outside the Piccadilly branch for a slow and enjoyable afternoon in Central London.

63–97 Kensington High Street, W8 5SE.
020 7368 4500
www.wholefoodsmarket.co.uk
High Street Kensington Tube.
Branches: Piccadilly Circus W1B 5AR, Richmond TW9 1AB, plus four more locations across London.

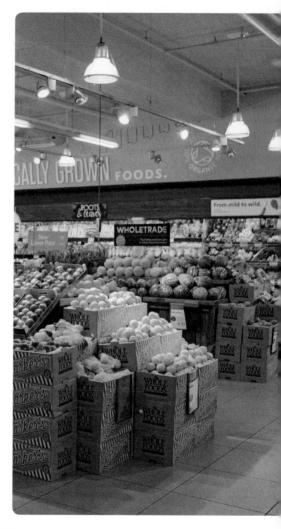

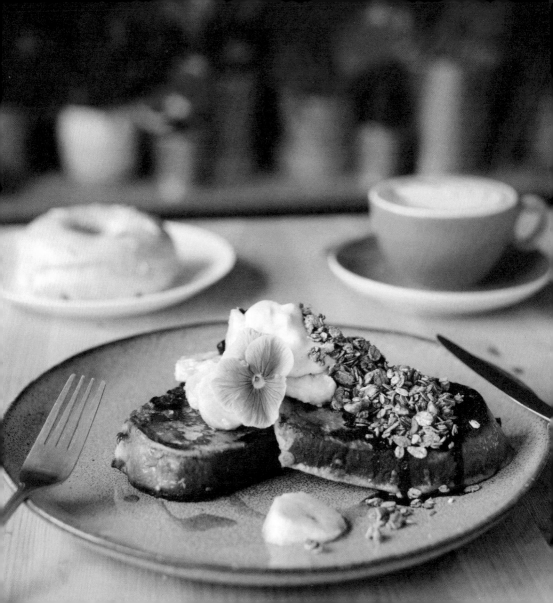

SWEET TREATS

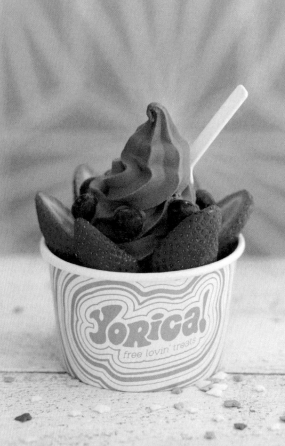

SWEET TREATS

Baking vegan is easier than you think. Keen sweet-toothed
vegans have come up with an answer for everything – from flaxseed 'eggs'
to cashew 'buttercream' – there's no need to make cake any other way.
Stepping up London's dessert game, the last decade has seen a huge
increase in vegan cake businesses as well as 'doughnutteries', cookie-makers
and patisseries. Gone are the days of sorbet being the only vegan option
for a third course. It's now common to see chocolate brownies, crumbles
and dairy-free ice cream even on chain-restaurant menus, as chefs respond
to the growing demand, and in this chapter you'll discover a mixture of
vegan-only brands plus popular non-vegan places serving up exceptional
vegan-friendly treats. Covering everything from raw, gluten-free cakes
to American-style pancake brunches, you'll be spoiled for choice the
next time you fancy something sweet.

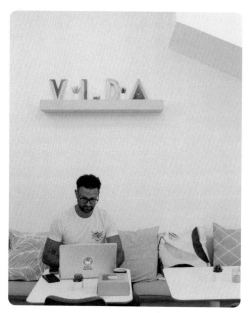

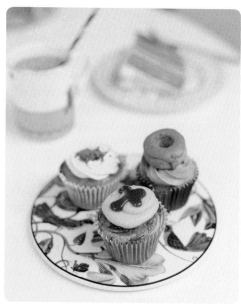

✤ VIDA BAKERY 100% VEGAN

The word vida means 'life' in Spanish, so Vida Bakery's name was chosen to reflect the brand and their ethos: a company full of life and a company that celebrates life. This, to founders Dani and Vane, means steering clear of animal-derived ingredients in their food to provide cruelty-free treats that suit all occasions. Known within the vegan community for their mini cupcakes and their extravagant customised cakes, Vida Bakery started out as a cake delivery company and now have their own café in Shoreditch. In the café, you'll find pastries, cinnamon buns and doughnuts alongside their cupcakes and larger cakes sold by the slice, encouraging cake connoisseurs to 'eat the rainbow'. The Vida team is also able to cater for gluten-free diets. Try the peanut-butter jelly and pretzel cupcake flavours, and don't leave Brick Lane without enjoying a slice of their notorious rainbow layer cake.

----

139 Brick Lane, E1 6SB.
07879 860 108
www.vidabakery.co.uk
Shoreditch High Street Overground.

VIDA - Bakery

139 BRICK LANE

139
Brick Lane

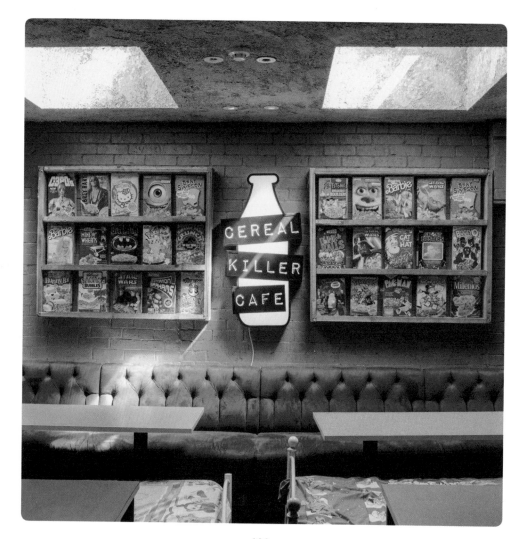

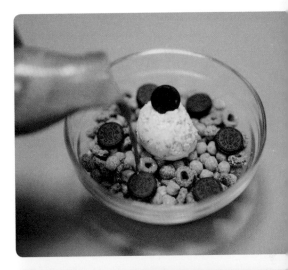

✤ CEREAL KILLER CAFE <u>VEGAN-FRIENDLY</u>

For a dose of 90s nostalgia, it has to be Cereal Killer. Twins Alan and Gary Keery opened the Brick Lane branch of this memorabilia-filled, cereal-based café in 2014, and the concept was so popular that they opened a second branch in Camden and then went global with further cafés in the Middle East. Selling international cereals in the form of cereal bowls and milkshakes, Cereal Killer have recently extended their vegan menu at the Shoreditch branch to include bowls served with oat milk, Cereal Milk Ice Cream made from soya-based ice cream soaked in Frosties, and shakes with oat milk and soya custard piled high with soya cream, cereal and sauce. There's also a vegan Pop Tart ice-cream sandwich and there are even savoury options including Arancheerio Balls: garlic risotto balls in a crispy Cheerio coating.

———

192A Brick Lane, E1 6SB.

020 3601 9100

www.cerealkillercafe.co.uk

Shoreditch High Street Overground.

Branches: Camden NW1 8AH.

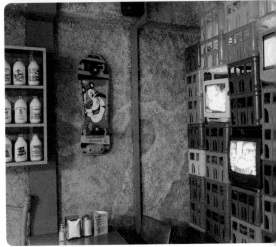

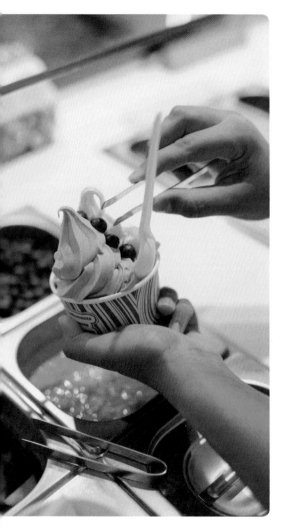

✤ YORICA! <u>100% VEGAN</u>

Allergy sufferers are often an afterthought at restaurants, but Yorica!'s purpose is to feed free-from desserts to the masses. There's no dairy, egg, gluten or nuts at their dessert parlour, and the menu spans vegan ice cream, fro-yo, shakes and crêpes. The ice-cream counter is home to classic flavours as well as more unusual ones, like bubblegum and violets, and toppings range from vegan marshmallows to berries to vegan gummy bears. You can even stuff your cone or tub with fluffy mini waffles before piling on free sprinkles – choose the 'Epic' tub size for maximum topping-space! You'll feel the 60s vibes flowing as soon as you enter. It's not unusual to make friends with other vegans in Yorica!'s Soho and Notting Hill hang-out spots, bonding over love for their Good Vibes Vanilla and Mellow Matcha fro-yo. It's free from, for everyone.

—

130 Wardour Street, W1F 8ZN.
020 7434 4370
www.yorica.com
Oxford Circus or Tottenham Court Road Tube.

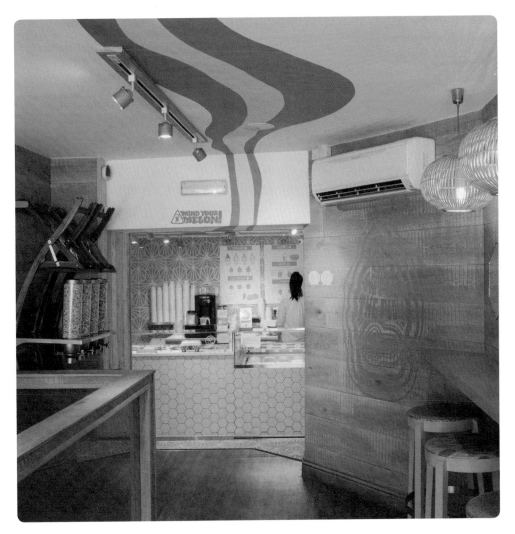

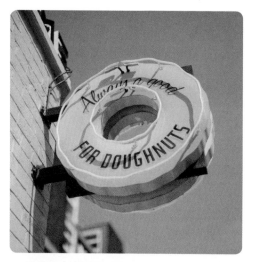

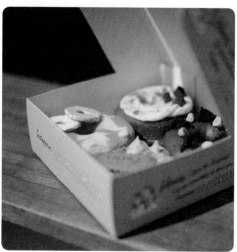

✤ DOUGHNUT TIME VEGAN-FRIENDLY

Some vegan doughnuts are baked instead of fried. Some are sugar-free. Some, even, are raw. Not so at Doughnut Time – this chain creates extravagant doughnut flavours, heavy with toppings and too pretty not to upload on Instagram. While most of their doughnuts are made with butter and milk, they've always got an impressive selection of vegan doughnuts, and the menu changes frequently. Recent flavours include Pump Up The Jam, with raspberry plum jam and cinnamon sugar, and the Cornelius Fudge, with a chocolate vegan glaze, topped with vegan brownies and toasted hazelnuts. It's also good to know that Doughnut Time's creations are fried in vegetable oil and contain no trans fats, and the doughnuts are delivered fresh to their stores each day. It's always a good time for these sweet snacks!

—

96 Shaftesbury Avenue, W1D 5ED.
020 3940 0594
www.doughnuttime.co.uk
Leicester Square Tube.
Branches: Shoreditch EC1V 9HE, Notting Hill W11 2EE, plus seven more locations across London.

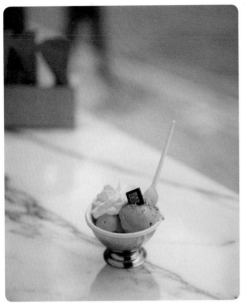
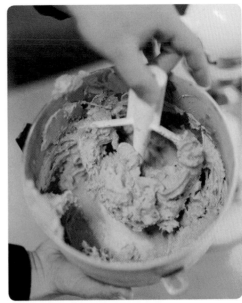

❖ CHIN CHIN LABS <u>VEGAN-FRIENDLY</u>

With a mission to create happy moments and inject fun into the lives of Londoners, Chin Chin have been hand-churning their ice cream with liquid nitrogen since opening their first store in Camden in 2010. Using organic ingredients where possible and producing in small batches, Chin Chin now serve their frozen treats at three locations: Camden, Soho and at Street Feast (Dinerama). Examples of vegan specials include Pandan flavour ice cream, Purple Violet and Pineapple and Habanero. The must-try topping is Chin Chin's Crack – a molten chocolate shell – but there's also pistachio and cardamom powder, raspberry sauce and handmade torched vegan marshmallows. As the menu changes weekly, you can check online to see which branches are serving flavours that most tickle your fancy – and check back week after week to discover new innovative creations and combinations.

—

49–50 Camden Lock Place, NW1 8AF.
www.chinchinicecream.com
Camden Town Tube.
Branches: Soho W1D 3DS, Shoreditch EC2A 3EJ.

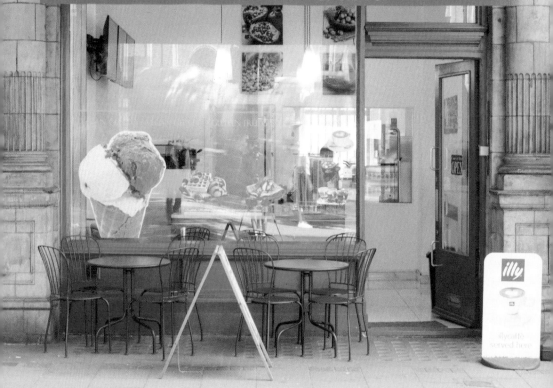

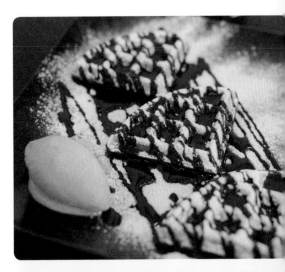

✤ PRIME GELATO <u>VEGAN-FRIENDLY</u>

While sorbets are usually vegan-friendly, it's harder to find a classic, creamy Italian gelato without dairy besides the odd dark chocolate flavour. Prime Gelato combats this with an entire range of vegan gelato: six flavours a day, with a changing menu designed by founder and gelato master Mirko Mazzone. The gelato base is made from water, vegetable milks and vegetable fats, and the different variations are created using ingredients such as fruit, cocoa and nuts – the seasons play a role in which foods are selected for the menu, and there's a strong focus on local ingredients too. Expect to explore flavours like mint chocolate chip, peanut and yuzu along with the typical dark chocolate – they even have a vegan cone that's gluten-free. And if you're after a vegan hot chocolate, Mirko has used his culinary expertise to craft one of the best dairy-free hot drinks in London.

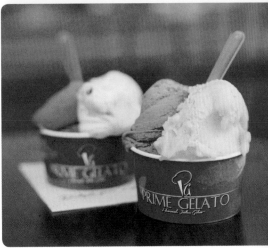

216 Shaftesbury Avenue, WC2H 8EB.
07840 803 338
www.primegelato.co.uk
Holborn or Tottenham Court Road Tube.

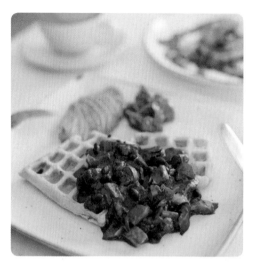

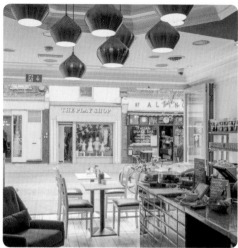

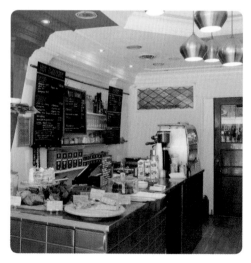

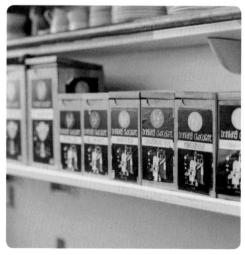

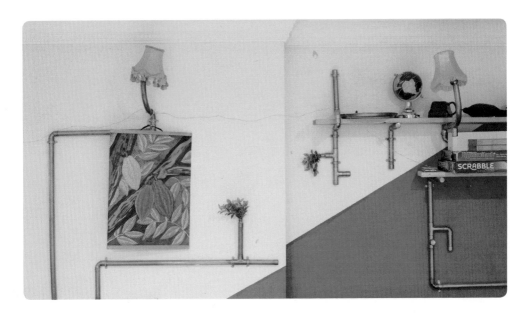

✤ JAZ & JUL'S <u>VEGAN-FRIENDLY</u>

Proving that chocolate doesn't need dairy to taste divine, Jaz & Jul's Chocolate House is home to award-winning hot chocolates made in on-site melted chocolate vats, plus an array of vegan cakes and a chocolate-inspired savoury menu. While not a completely vegan café, you'll find plenty of vegan cakes on the counter that you can tuck into while having a moment to yourself in one of their cosy armchairs with a book and a hot drink – it's like your living room away from home. What's more, the café hosts a chocolate-themed bottomless brunch on the weekends, with both savoury and sweet vegan options, unlimited Prosecco or special cocoa-influenced breakfast cocktails, plus bottomless chocolate sauce. And if you're still able to think about chocolate after London's most chocolatey two-hour dining experience, you can always buy their hot chocolates to take home or to give as gifts.

----

1 Chapel Market, London N1 9EZ.

020 3583 4375

www.jazandjuls.co.uk

Angel Tube.

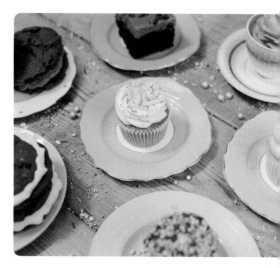

✤ MS. CUPCAKE 100% VEGAN

Ms. Cupcake is London's original, classic vegan bakery. You'll find a counter full of cupcakes, cookies and layer cakes plus sandwiches and other savoury foods at the Brixton bakery, alongside take-home items like vegan ice-cream tubs and snack bars. This variety of quality products even prompted Ms. Cupcake to be awarded as Dot London's Best Independent Retailer in 2016. Not content with just feeding Londoners great vegan food, Ms. Cupcake herself – Mellissa Morgan – has gone one step further by writing her own cookbook to share her knowledge of vegan baking and encourage others to leave dairy and egg out of their cakes. Ms. Cupcake is known for its icing-heavy approach, crowning cupcakes with sweet swirls of flavours including red velvet and salted caramel. Many of their creations are also made without gluten, tying in with the bakery's vision that everybody deserves great cake regardless of their dietary requirements.

---

408 Coldharbour Lane, SW9 8LF.
020 3086 8933
www.mscupcake.co.uk
Brixton Tube.

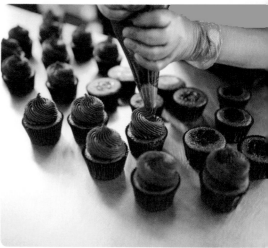

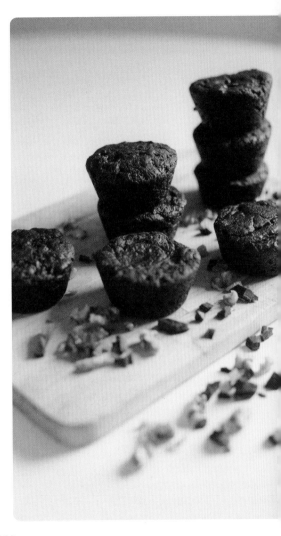

✤ COOKIE & BISCUIT <u>100% VEGAN</u>

Cookie & Biscuit started as a small-batch bakery in South London in 2013, as a way to satisfy founder Danae's sweet tooth with healthier alternatives that were free from egg and dairy. Using unrefined sugars and a variety of flours from gluten-free to spelt, the Cookie & Biscuit team now pride themselves on creating delicious bespoke cakes and brownies, for pick-up and delivery, that everyone can enjoy. Having traded at local farmers' markets and catering private events, Cookie & Biscuit have also launched sister brand The V Spot – under this name, you'll find yoga brunches and supper clubs in London, plus catering for weddings and events. Cookie & Biscuit are perhaps best known on the vegan scene for their brownie subscription boxes, which can be ordered online. Each month, they send out two different flavours of delicious fudgy brownie boxes all over the UK.

Events across London and deliveries across London and the UK (see website for details).

www.cookieandbiscuit.com

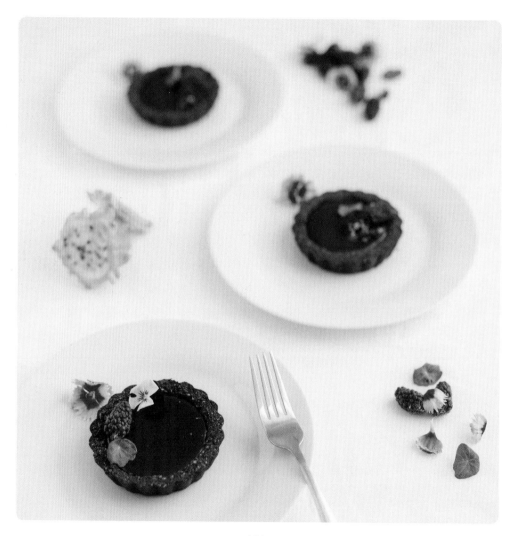

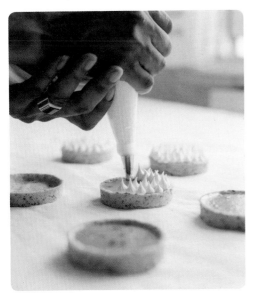
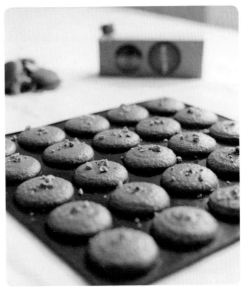

✤ ORGANIC LIVITY 100% VEGAN

If you're looking to appreciate every flavour in a dish, head to one of Organic Livity's foodie events, or have their raw cakes and patisserie treats delivered to your door across London. Originating from the luscious Caribbean island of Martinique, artisan chef Sidney draws on his knowledge of so-called 'indigenous' ingredients to craft truly unique creations including raw cakes, macarons, gluten-free artisan breads and raw doughnuts. For a raw cake with a difference, savour the flavours of the Afro Me Vogue: camu camu, cacao, blueberry, cherry, blue algae, cacao butter, pistachio, quinoa and vanilla pod from Reunion Island. There are also colourful, eggless macarons and cinnamon cookies sweetened with molasses — and for a romantic treat, try the Aphrodisiac Secrete Tarte with an Irish moss raspberry jelly and a French cacao ganache. Organic Livity offer dining experiences across London, including supper clubs, afternoon teas and yoga brunches.

Events and deliveries across London
(see website for details).
www.organiclivityco.com

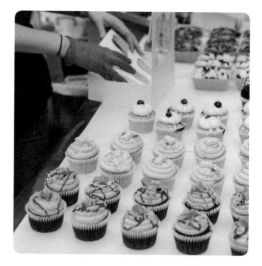

✤ RUBYS OF LONDON 100% VEGAN

Talented baker Ruby came to realise her passion for making visually stunning free-from treats as a result of a childhood dairy and egg allergy. Feeling uninspired by the dairy- and egg-free options greeting her at birthday parties as a girl, Ruby turned things around to inspire others that free-from food can be sumptuous while looking as good as it tastes. After many years of vegan baking, the Rubys of London weekend Greenwich Market stall opened and people travelled miles to try Ruby's freshly baked cupcakes, doughnuts and more. The products change weekly, with an aim to continuously develop and experiment with artistic and delicious creations – this dedication landed Ruby the 2013 British Baker Product Innovation Award. On top of the Greenwich stall, the full Rubys of London range is available online to deliver across Greater London – don't miss the classic carrot cake and the almost-too-pretty-to-eat doughnuts.

———

Greenwich Market, SE10 9HZ.
020 8858 6618
www.rubysoflondon.com
Greenwich DLR.

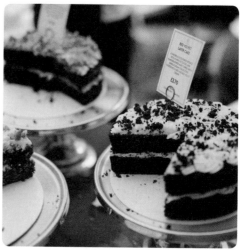

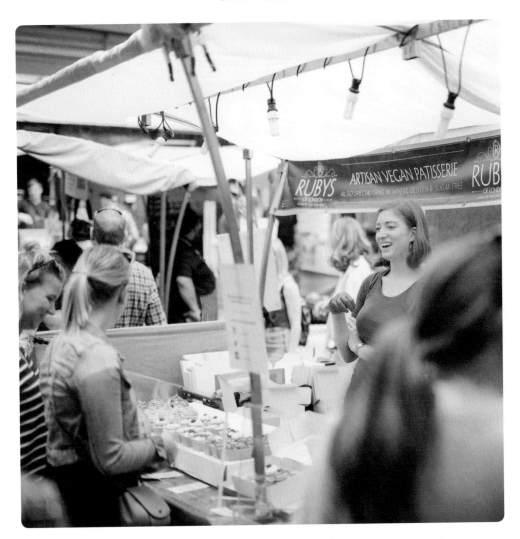

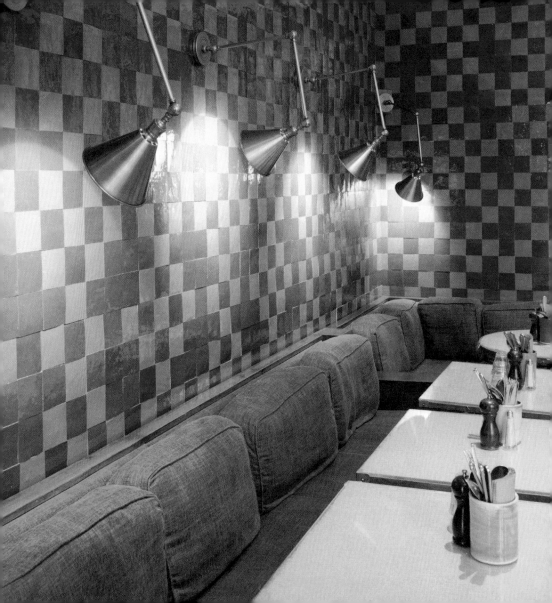

CAFÉ CULTURE

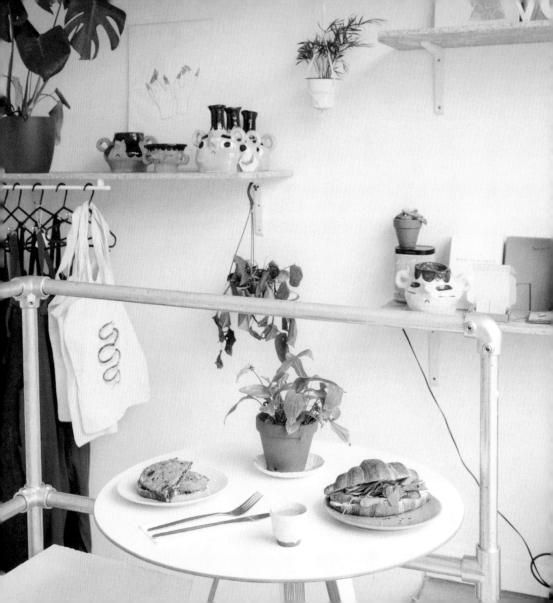

CAFÉ CULTURE

From west to east, London is home to hundreds of wile-away-your-time, cosy coffee houses and sandwich spots, from the well-known and bustling to the hidden local gems. The capital's café culture is eclectic, homely and always welcoming – whether it's your first or twentieth visit, you can grab a flat white and a croissant and make yourself comfortable. So what happens to the café experience when you minus the dairy milk from your hot chocolate and the eggs from your brunch? Not a lot, actually. The majority of vegans used to eat and drink the same way as everybody else and, as a result, there's now foaming oat milk and tofu scramble to step in and transform those nostalgic café treats – so you can continue enjoying the best that London has to offer, just in vegan form. Pain au chocolat, anyone?

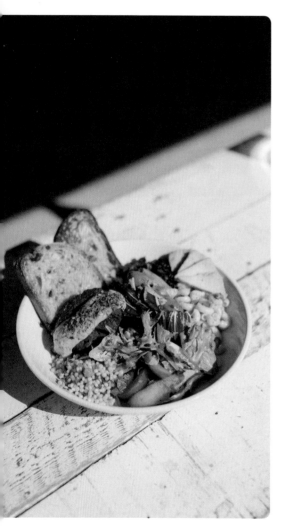

✤ BLACK CAT 100% VEGAN

For some of the best value-for-money food in London, look no further than Black Cat in Hackney. The portions are generous and the prices are happily affordable. A busy hotspot for East London locals, you'll find vegans browsing the offerings of reusable coffee cups and an array of chocolate bars from Black Cat's shelves while waiting for their food to be served. Many of these items are sourced locally, complementing the locally roasted coffee and supporting small businesses. On the menu, you'll find staples such as Black Cat's seitan and soya mince patty with vegan mayo and a locally made bun, a barbecue tofu sandwich served on a sourdough ciabatta and their chickpea flour pancakes served with roasted vegetables. On top of this, there are daily specials, fruity soya milkshakes and pastries and cakes so good you'll end up buying extra to take home.

76A Clarence Road, E5 8HB.
020 8985 7091
www.blackcatcafe.co.uk
Hackney Central Overground.

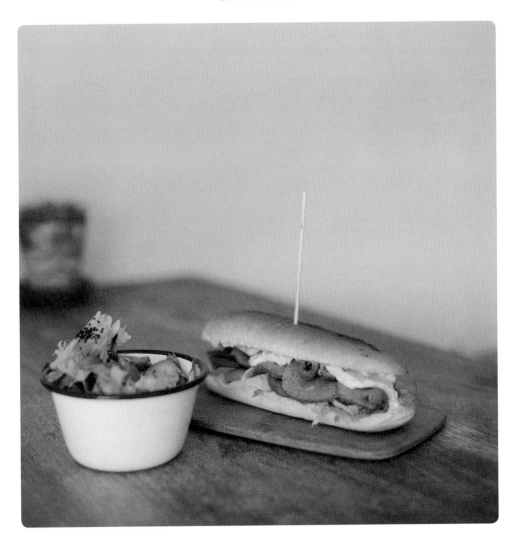

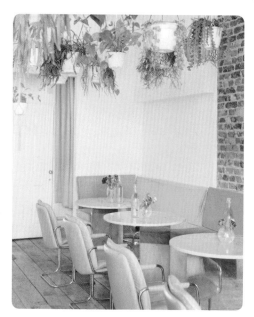

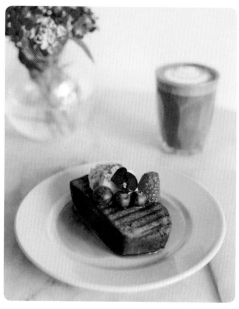

❖ PALM VAULTS <u>VEGAN-FRIENDLY</u>

This pastel paradise will take you on vacation to 1980s Miami with its mint green and baby pink interior, complete with hanging plants and tropical prints. Listed by *Time Out* as one of the prettiest places to get coffee in London, you won't feel alone undertaking a full photoshoot with your red velvet latte (coloured with beetroot) and your wedge of pink layer cake. But Palm Vaults is more than just a pretty face. On their fully vegetarian menu, they offer some of the best vegan cheese melted sandwiches in London – the Firecracker melt is a force to be reckoned with. For your coffee, choose from a range of plant milks – and their takeaway coffee cups are equally as photogenic as the decor. Bring your camera, your dog and your appetite – but leave your MacBook at home; there's a no-laptop rule as otherwise none of us would ever leave this 80s haven.

—

411 Mare Street, E8 1HY.

www.palmvaults.com

Hackney Central Overground.

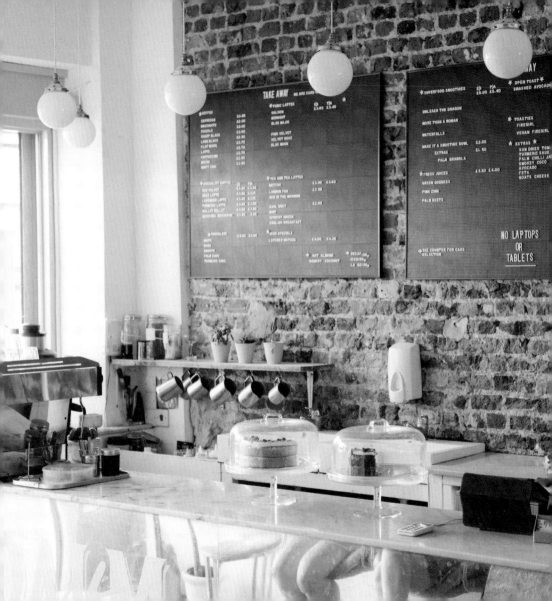

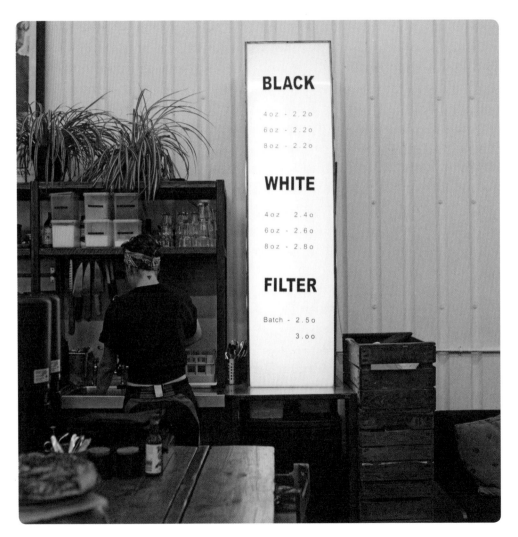

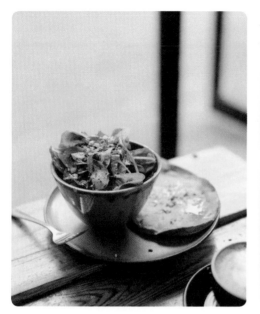
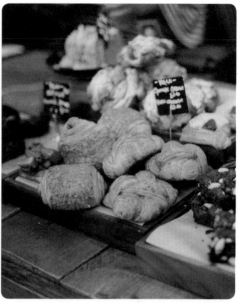

✤ I WILL KILL AGAIN <u>VEGAN-FRIENDLY</u>

What do you get when you cross biker culture, the occult and single-origin coffee? The answer is nestled under the railway arches between Hackney and Homerton – I Will Kill Again, a café situated inside Dark Arts Coffee roastery. The café is not only unique in its decor – think Satan's Sadists and The Blood on Satan's Claw movie posters combined with welcoming sofas and spider plants. It's also a rare find in that it serves a mostly vegan menu with a couple of meat options – not exclusively vegan, but flipping things the other way around from a regular café menu. Dark Arts' coffee is hailed as being some of the best speciality coffee in London, and their brunch is on everyone's must-try list. Go for a vegan breakfast muffin and a couple of their pastries (berry Danish, anyone?), and tuck into a vegan chocolate waffle on the weekend menu.

—

Arch 216, 27A Ponsford Street, E9 6JU.
020 3774 0131
www.facebook.com/iwillkillagain
Homerton or Hackney Central Overground.

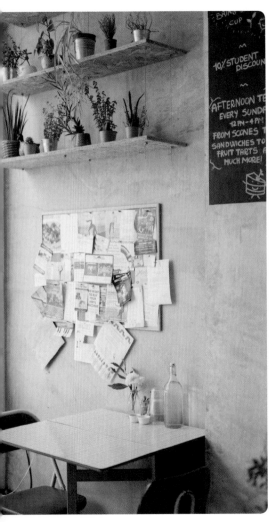

✤ LELE'S <u>100% VEGAN</u>

Lele's is everything a café should be: the team serve great coffee, they encourage sitting and having a 'good natter', they love dogs, and the combination of the naturally light and bright space and the homely setup creates an atmosphere as welcoming as the people. There are so many 'right times' to visit Lele's. Breakfast is a must, with the Sweet Little Things selection encompassing plain and filled croissants, pain au raisins, peanut-butter on toast and more – all freshly baked. For lunch, try the Happy Zz open toast with scrambled tofu and avocado – named after founder Valentina's rescue dog, who you might bump into at the café. Then there's the afternoon tea: one Sunday each month, you can sample all the vegan patisserie treats that Lele's offer, along with a selection of teas. If you can't make it to Clapton, Lele's trade regularly at markets across London.

----

50 Lower Clapton Road, E5 0RN.
www.leleslondon.com
Hackney Downs, Hackney Central or
Homerton Overground.

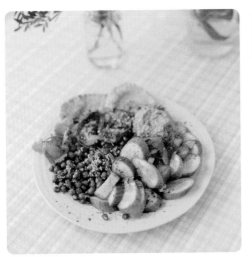

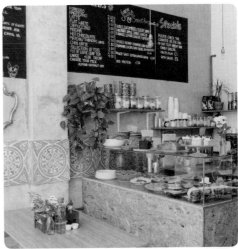

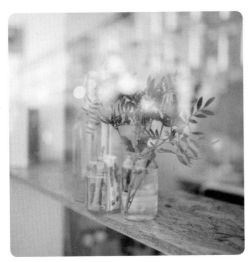

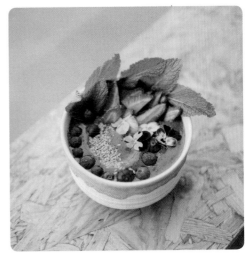

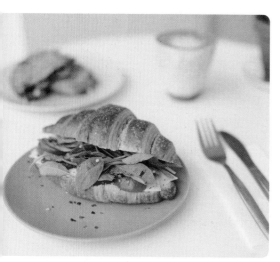

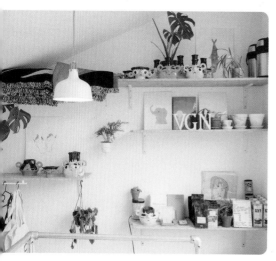

✤ UNRIPE BANANA 100% VEGAN

For a full-to-the-brim brunch in East London, visit Unripe Banana just across from Hackney City Farm. It looks like a small space from the outside, but head downstairs to explore more: you might find an exhibition going on, a workshop or one of the many events Unripe Banana hosts underneath the café. Upstairs is where the food is at, and the must-try dish is the savoury pancakes stack. Colourful deep-red and yellow fluffy pancakes, oozing with speciality Kinda Co. cheese sauce, are topped with avocado and seeds and finished with a handful of chopped greens. Max out with a tomato and vegan cheese croissant and sip on a hot drink – Unripe Banana take pride in their coffee, and you can opt for Oatly Barista or choose from almond, cashew or coconut Mylkman. Best enjoyed with a sticky chocolate brownie. Everything's vegan, so brunch your heart out.

———

Unit 7, 268 Hackney Road, E2 7SJ.
www.unripebanana.co.uk
Hoxton or Cambridge Heath Overground.

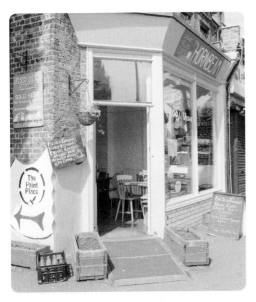

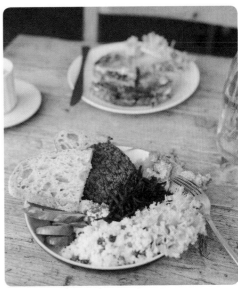

✤ HORNBEAM CAFÉ <u>100% VEGAN</u>

Brightening up a typically busy East London road, the Hornbeam Café is a tidy, community-linked, zero-waste café. It's high up on the list in terms of ethical eateries and exclusively serves vegan food, with local, organic and fairly traded ingredients to the best of their ability. The café uses fresh fruit and vegetables from their local growing co-operative, Organiclea, which runs a weekly stall outside the café in the spring. The Hornbeam serves a range of meals, including their well-known vegan Sunday roast and, if that doesn't tickle your fancy, their brunch or selection of freshly baked cakes should go down well. It's hard to knock Hornbeam Café's approach to business and their community – promoting sustainable living and inspiring people to think about ethical resource management. Operating alongside the community and run for the community, Hornbeam Café is a flag-bearer for ethical and local food.

—

458 Hoe Street, E17 9AH.
020 8558 6880
www.hornbeam.org.uk
Walthamstow Central Tube.

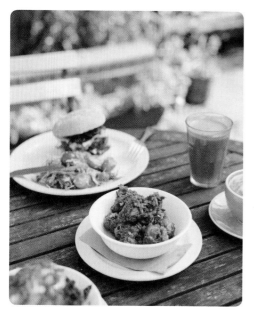
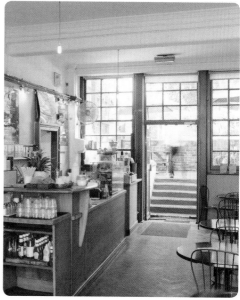

❖ THE GALLERY CAFÉ 100% VEGAN

Bethnal Green is an area so rich in East London history, yet untouched by tourists when compared with the likes of neighbouring Shoreditch and Stratford. The Gallery Café is part of St Margaret's House, a charity supporting community, creativity and wellbeing for more than 120 years. When the sun is shining, feast on pancakes with seasonal fruit on the outdoor terrace and, in the winter, warm up with a chai latte while listening to live music. One other must-try item on The Gallery Cafe's menu is their Full English: vegan sausages, scrambled tofu, fried potatoes, sautéed kale, mushrooms, tomatoes, homemade baked beans and sourdough toast. Start at the Stairway To Heaven memorial at Bethnal Green station, enjoy Bethnal Green Gardens and then wander up to the V&A Museum of Childhood and finish off with a trip to The Gallery Café for a quieter day out, escaping the crowds.

21 Old Ford Road, E2 9PL.

020 8980 2092

www.stmargaretshouse.org.uk/gallerycafe

Bethnal Green Tube.

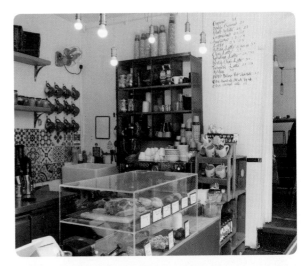

✤ LLS CAFÉ <u>VEGAN-FRIENDLY</u>

LLS is the kind of local gem that's almost too good to share. Entering the small and bustling café, you'll eye up the cake counter and make a mental note of at least three cakes to take away with you on the way out. With even their toast homemade, LLS's ethos is that real food should be the foundation of a good diet regardless of fitness goals, and so they work to feed Londoners healthy food that tastes great. Situated at the less busy end of Heath Street in Hampstead, this is the perfect place to spend a Saturday brunch session complete with their signature LLS buckwheat pancakes served with coconut cream, chia jam, banana and berries. Bring your dog and follow brunch with a walk up the road to the beautiful Hampstead Heath.

—

95–97 Heath Street, NW3 6SS.

020 7794 8600

www.llscafe.com

Hampstead Tube.

Branches: Waterloo SE1 7NJ, Lancaster Gate W2 3EL

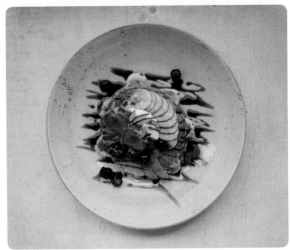

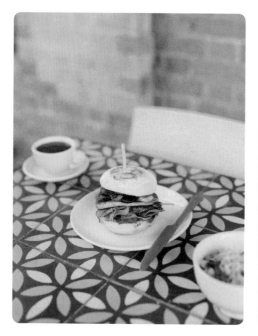

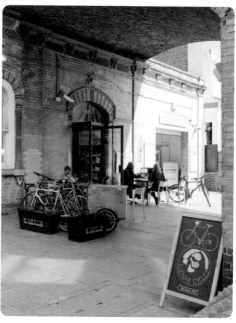

✤ THE FIELDS BENEATH 100% VEGAN

The Fields Beneath has been a popular café since 2012, serving coffee and mum's cakes to the people of Kentish Town. Their story is particularly special, with one team member becoming vegan and helping the whole business make the switch. The café spent weeks being 'out of ham', and then flyers appeared explaining why there'd soon be no dairy milk served in their coffees anymore. They went completely vegan on Mother's Day 2017 and, with resounding support from both vegans and old regulars impressed by the still-delicious food and drink, the team are planning to open more sites soon. Visit The Fields Beneath for stuffed croissants, sausage rolls, cake and delicious Oatly-brewed coffee – and get ready to visit time and time again.

—

52A Prince of Wales Road, Kentish Town, NW5 3LN.
020 7424 8838
www.thefieldsbeneath.com
Kentish Town Overground.

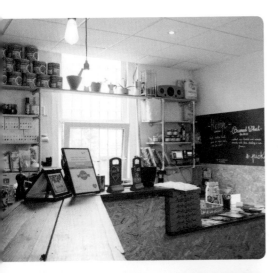

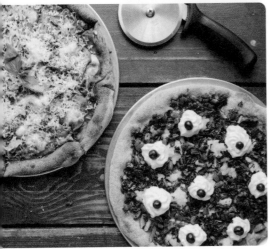

✣ PICKYWOPS 100% VEGAN

At PickyWops' vegan pizzeria, the base is just as important as the topping, with five bases each changing the flavour experience entirely. The blue-green spirulina base is a healthy choice, packed with vitamins and low in cholesterol. For a richer flavour, try the toasted wheat mix minced coarsely with white flour. Watching your macros? Try the kamut with Khorasan wheat – kamut flour is a good source of protein. Finally, if you've tried everything from turmeric shots to golden lattes, it's time to level up with a turmeric-based pizza. With eighteen pizza and calzone options involving intriguing names like the Ravenous Lumberjack and the Vegan Victory, plus lots of extras available, the combinations at PickyWops are almost endless. Whether you're after something light and green, or heavy with vegan salami and sausage, PickyWops has a pizza perfect for you.

20–22 Peckham Rye, SE15 4JR.
07427 076 525
www.pickywops.com
Peckham Rye Overground.

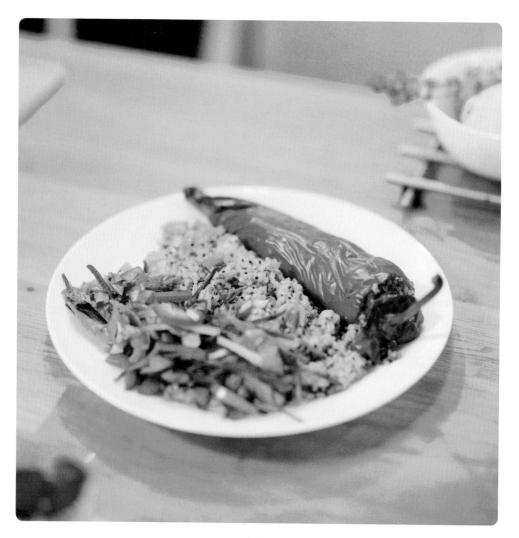

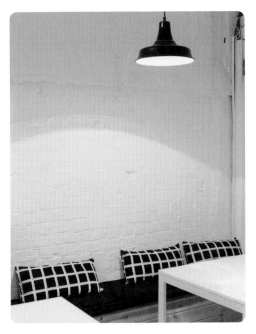
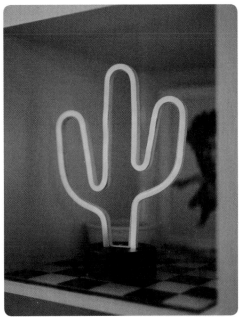

✤ DESERTED CACTUS <u>100% VEGAN</u>

Forget chia-seed bliss balls and gluten-free raw cheesecakes – the only balls of bliss you'll find at Deserted Cactus are café owner Esme's plantain dumplings, golden brown and with just the right balance of sweet and spice. Esme, AKA food blogger London Afro Vegan, will make sure you leave stuffed with tasty plant-based food that you could replicate at home – many of her recipes are on her YouTube channel, and it's this accessibility that makes Deserted Cactus such a likeable café.

There's no official menu, but expect to be fed dishes along the lines of Mac No Cheese (which makes a regular appearance), stuffed baked sweet peppers with tomato quinoa, cauliflower steaks and Esme's Southern-fried jackfruit burger. New food every day means it'd be silly not to return to the Deserted Cactus – go with an empty stomach.

Units 23 & 25 Holdrons Arcade, 135A Rye Lane, SE15 4ST.
www.facebook.com/desertedcactus
Peckham Rye Overground.

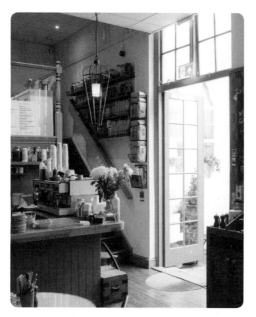

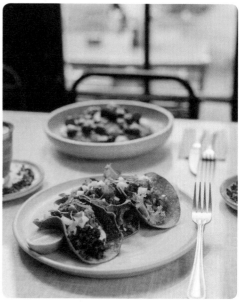

✤ FARM GIRL <u>VEGAN-FRIENDLY</u>

An idyllic place to catch up with a friend over a Butterfly Matcha, Farm Girl offers brunches and lunches that are both hearty and healthy – Australian founder and ex-farm girl Rose wanted to build a menu based on nutritious staples like homemade granola, toast and porridge. With three branches in West and Central London, the cafés merge country and city vibes. The Chelsea all-day restaurant is a sight to behold – the back half of the establishment has a transparent roof, allowing daylight to pour through the leaves of plants lining the tops of the walls and down onto your acai bowl. Or if you'd rather refuel with a coconut 'bacon' sandwich after a workout, head to the Farm Girl café within Sweaty Betty in Soho, where you can workout, shop and enjoy a slice of avo toast and pomegranate all in a day's work.

—

9 Park Walk, SW10 0AJ.
020 3674 7359
www.thefarmgirl.co.uk
South Kensington or Fulham Broadway Tube.
Branches: Notting Hill W11 3DB, Soho W1F 9QG.

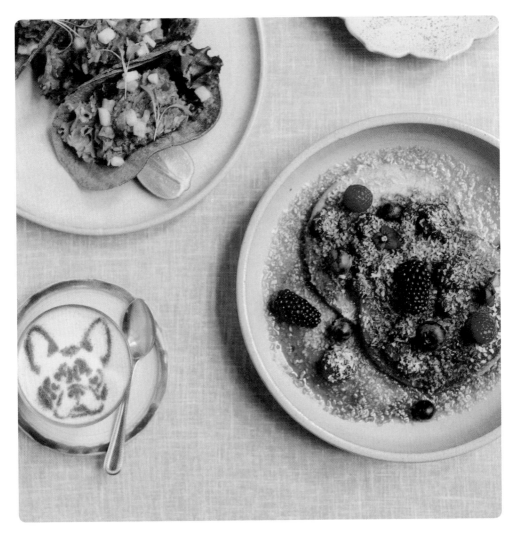

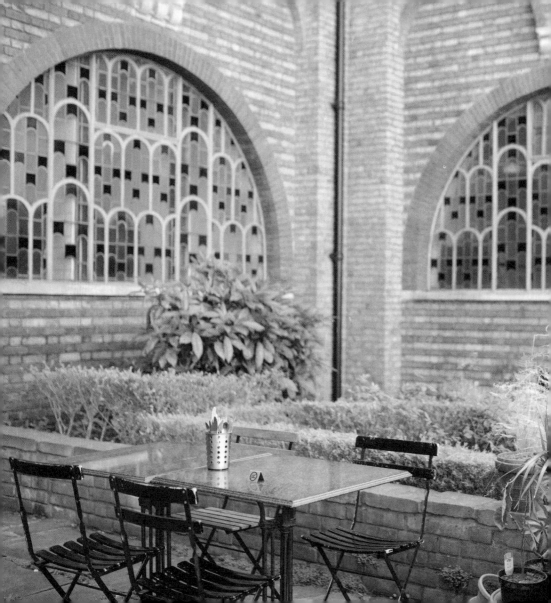

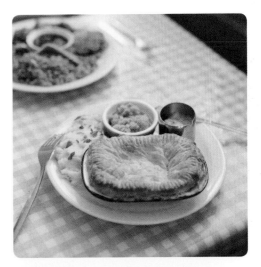

✤ CAFE VAN GOGH <u>100% VEGAN</u>

Brixton has Cafe Van Gogh founder Steve Clarke to thank for creating one of the most charismatic eateries in London, and making it one of the most ethical at that. Entering the lower floor, a winding staircase laced with colourful lights leads you up to a cosy, exposed-brick setting. Paying homage to Van Gogh's *Starry Night*, the raised ceiling is painted midnight blue and dotted with white and yellow. The menu includes vegan improvements on nostalgic comfort food – you might find a seitan Guinness pie, as well as the traditional Sunday roast based around a nut roast wellington and veggies. Or choose from the team's travel-inspired options, such as the popular jerk plantain with butternut chilli and caramelised pineapple. And the best bit of all? Cafe Van Gogh is a non-profit restaurant. Profits are reinvested into dedicated programmes within the local community that provide on-the-job training and food nutrition workshops.

----

88 Brixton Road, SW9 6BE.
07546 966 554
www.cafevangogh.co.uk
Oval Tube.

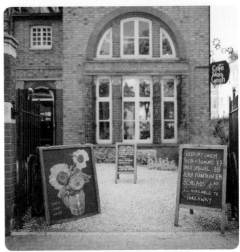

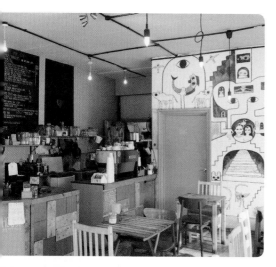

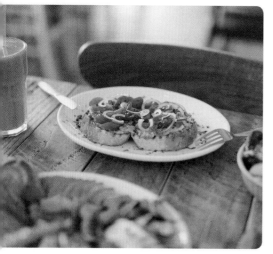

☘ THE GREENHOUSE DEPTFORD

<u>VEGAN-FRIENDLY</u>

The Greenhouse Deptford caters for a range of dietary requirements and, while it's not exclusively vegan, they serve up plant-based options as well as gluten-sensitive and low-carb options. The Greenhouse focuses on keeping their menu simple while supporting local, eco-friendly businesses. It's all about the details – from their ethically sourced coffee to the community-created murals on their walls. From their approach to compostable packaging to their locally made cola, The Greenhouse has left no stone unturned, creating a café which serves the community with sustainability in mind. When it comes to the food, you can go down the traditional route with a fresh-fruit-laden granola, or take their refreshing alternative to a full English for breakfast and try their Mediterranean platter mix with hummus, aubergine, avocado and a mixed salad.

----

481 New Cross Road, SE14 6TA.
www.greenhousedeptford.co.uk
New Cross Overground.

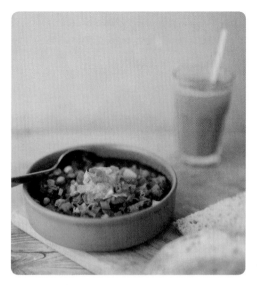
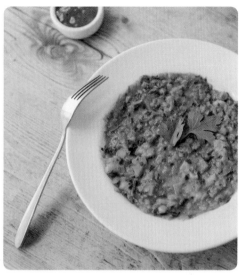

❧ LE PAIN QUOTIDIEN <u>VEGAN-FRIENDLY</u>

From West End shows to shopping mall sprees, Le Pain Quotidien is the perfect break from any day out – its 25 London eateries are dotted all the way from Shepherd's Bush to Canary Wharf. The easy-to-read menu marks vegan-friendly options with a carrot symbol, so you can clearly see all their delicious plant-based options from brunch to desserts and specials. Serious about breakfast, you'll find plenty of flavoursome dishes at LPQ, including the Detox Breakfast Bowl with coconut yoghurt, nuts, seeds, fresh fruit and agave syrup and a classic avocado toast with citrus cumin salt, topped with seeds. The Chilli Sin Carne with soya soured cream and the Lebanese Mezze are popular choices for a hearty lunch, and Le Pain Quotidien's Cocoa and Pear Cake won the Best Vegan Cake award from PETA in 2016. The London Bridge restaurant is particularly stunning, set in a warehouse-style building complete with a glass roof.

—

212 Fulham Road, SW10 9PJ.
020 3823 4510
www.lepainquotidien.co.uk
Gloucester Road Tube.
Branches: Covent Garden WC2E 8RF, London Bridge SE1 9AG, plus 22 other locations across London.

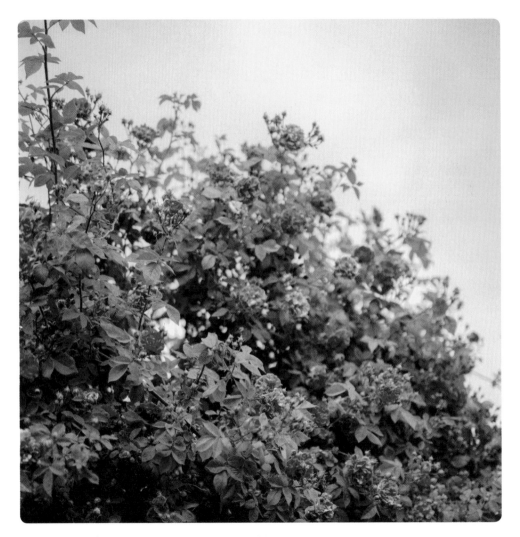

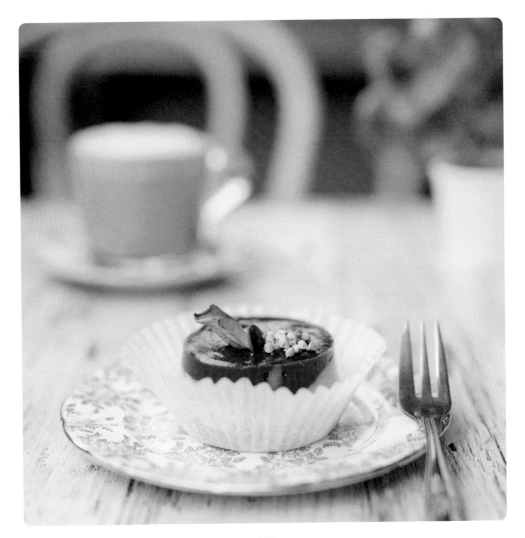

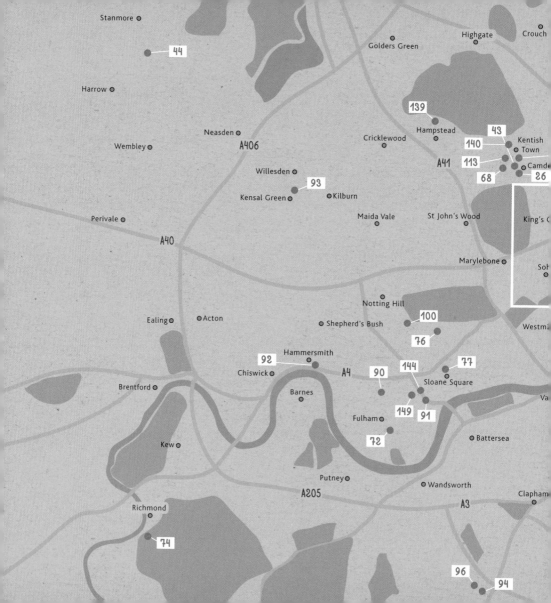

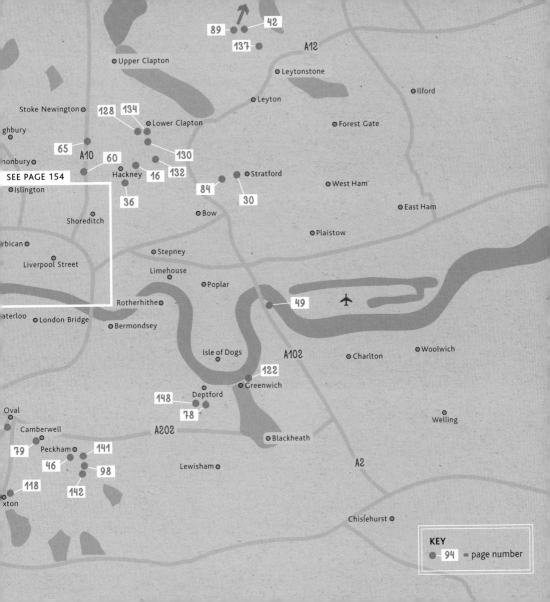

89
42
137
A12
Upper Clapton
Leytonstone
Ilford
Stoke Newington
Leyton
128 134
Lower Clapton
Forest Gate
ghbury
65
A10
130
onbury
60
Hackney
16 132
84
Stratford
SEE PAGE 154
36
30
West Ham
Islington
East Ham
Shoreditch
Bow
rbican
Plaistow
Stepney
Liverpool Street
Limehouse
aterloo
London Bridge
Poplar
Rotherhithe
49
Bermondsey
Isle of Dogs
A102
Charlton
Woolwich
Greenwich
122
Oval
148
Deptford
Camberwell
78
Welling
79
Peckham
141
A202
46
98
Lewisham
A2
118
142
xton
Blackheath
Chislehurst

KEY

94 = page number

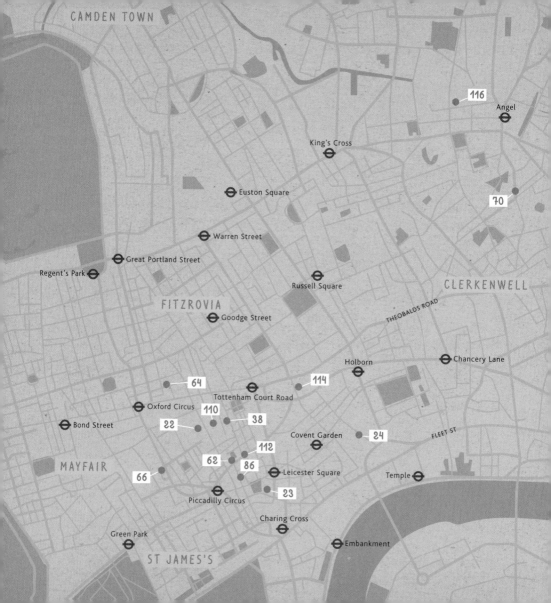

CAMDEN TOWN

116

Angel

King's Cross

Euston Square

70

Warren Street

Great Portland Street

Regent's Park

CLERKENWELL

Russell Square

FITZROVIA

THEOBALDS ROAD

Goodge Street

Holborn

Chancery Lane

64

114

Tottenham Court Road

Oxford Circus

110

38

22

Bond Street

Covent Garden

24

FLEET ST

112

MAYFAIR

62

86

66

Leicester Square

Temple

23

Piccadilly Circus

Charing Cross

Green Park

Embankment

ST JAMES'S

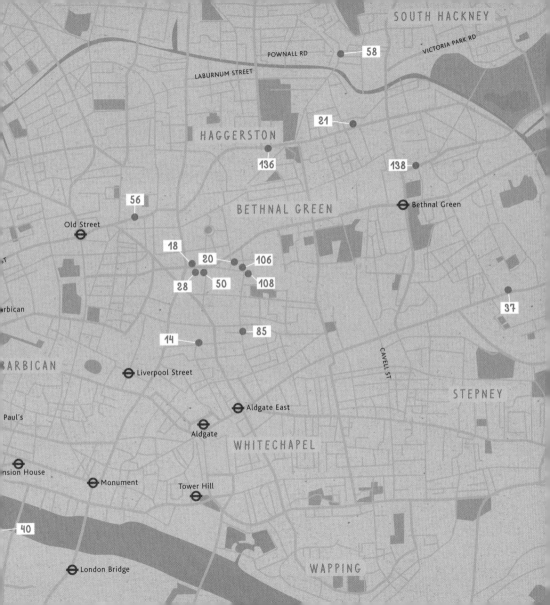

INDEX

Italics indicate branches.

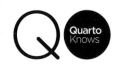

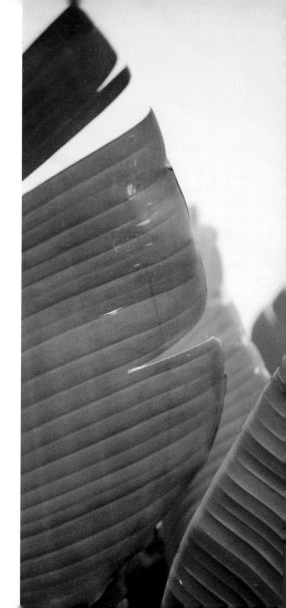

Brimming with creative inspiration, how-to projects and useful information to enrich your everyday life, Quarto Knows is a favourite destination for those pursuing their interests and passions. Visit our site and dig deeper with our books into your area of interest: Quarto Creates, Quarto Cooks, Quarto Homes, Quarto Lives, Quarto Drives, Quarto Explores, Quarto Gifts, or Quarto Kids.

First published in 2019 by White Lion Publishing, an imprint of The Quarto Group.
The Old Brewery, 6 Blundell Street
London, N7 9BH,
United Kingdom
T (0)20 7700 6700 F (0)20 7700 8066
www.QuartoKnows.com

A catalogue record for this book is available from the British Library.

ISBN 978 0 71124 011 7

Ebook ISBN 978 0 71124 012 4

10 9 8 7 6 5 4 3 2

Design by Sarah Pyke

Printed in China

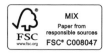

MIX
Paper from
responsible sources
FSC® C008047